THE GLUTEN, WHEAT & DAIRY FREE COOKBOOK

The Gluten, Wheat & Dairy Free Cookbook

Antoinette Savill

In Association with
Wellfoods (UK) Ltd.
Makers of
Gluten Free Flour

Thorsons

Thorsons
An Imprint of HarperCollins*Publishers*
77–85 Fulham Palace Road,
Hammersmith, London W6 8JB

The Thorsons website address is:
www.thorsons.com

Published by Thorsons 2000
1 3 5 7 9 10 8 6 4 2

© Antoinette Savill 2000
Photography by John Turner and Dave King

Antoinette Savill asserts the moral right to
be identified as the author of this work

A catalogue record for this book
is available from the British Library

ISBN 0 7225 4027 2

Printed and bound in Great Britain

Contents

Acknowledgements

First of all I would like to thank the most important person in my life, Stephen Lawrence, who has constantly guided, supported and advised me. I would also like to thank Sir Charles Jessell for his advice and encouragement, and Wanda Whiteley for encouraging me to concoct lots of recipes for those with a sweet tooth! Finally, I'd like to thank everyone who has helped put this book together.

Foreword

Diet is a four letter word, and it is often accompanied by a five letter word: gloom. This is a book to dispel any such ideas of despondency. It is about celebration. There is no reason why people with food intolerance should not enjoy their meals as much as anyone else, provided they follow the advice of people like Antoinette Savill.

She, and I, and, it is estimated, about sixty percent of the world's population, suffer from sensitivity to certain items in their diet. So this book should have a wide appeal to anyone who wants to have a social occasion with a meal that does not leave them, or their guests, feeling ill afterwards.

By careful manipulation, it is always possible to avoid one's worst food antagonists. However, Antoinette Savill makes it a pleasure. Jack Sprat *and* his wife would both be able to come to her parties – and to yours, if you read this book and act upon it. I recommend you to have it in your kitchen, and you will be ready to receive them.

Charles Jessell
Chairman of Governors, 1997-8
The Institute for Optimum Nutrition

Introduction

For many years, people have known that stress, pollution and junk food take their toll on our systems. The result of this onslaught is that more and more people are being diagnosed as suffering from food intolerances or dietary problems, and are being advised to follow bland, unappetizing diets. Having experienced the misery of such advice and the monotony and frustration of a restrictive diet, I decided to develop these recipes to prove that it is possible to eat exciting food and stay healthy.

The purpose of this cookbook is to allow those with food intolerances to entertain family and friends on all occasions and throughout the various celebrations of the year, giving everyone such delicious food that none will even realize that the ingredients are slightly different. The idea then is to make entertaining, be it a children's tea party or a simple picnic in the garden, a relaxing, fun and sociable few hours for everyone – including the cook!

My passion for food comes, essentially, from the intoxicating Mediterranean flavours: ripe and heady smells of fresh herbs, fruit and vegetables that are piled up on market stalls and wicker baskets, displayed casually but always looking glorious and in harmony with their surroundings. Not for me the regimented piles of perfect supermarket fruit and vegetables that all too often have no perceptible aroma but only a flaccid dullness evocative of nothing except the mysteries of science. This cosmopolitan collection of recipes, although at heart European, also has a sprinkling of oriental and Asian influences, whose intriguing ingredients are now available all over the world.

Food intolerance is, by its nature, a complex subject and no two people experience exactly the same intolerance. While nearly all the recipes in this book are dairy or wheat free and so helpful to IBS and ME/chronic fatigue sufferers as well as others, there are plenty of gluten-free recipes for coeliacs. Please remember that other ingredients included in the recipe may not be suitable for individual intolerance. If you are new to this challenging game of food avoidance, the table on page 266 will reassure you. It is important, however, that you do not try to diagnose or treat yourself: if you are having problems with foods or liquids do seek the advice and help of a good nutritionist, doctor or homeopathic practitioner. This book will help you to avoid certain foods while still letting you enjoy food, but will not cure your intolerance.

Many of the recipes in this book were once 'conventional' ones that that were totally hostile to my dietary needs. Having decided that I enjoyed them too much to give them up, I set about replacing the conventional ingredients with appropriate substitutes – for instance, sunflower and soya products replaced dairy, while corn and rice products replaced starch and cereals. Now, having familiarized myself with the fundamental problems associated with juggling ingredients, I can safely and quickly prepare menus to suit even the most restrictive of diets. This process of substituting ingredients is not only of benefit to those with food intolerances: medical opinion is now that we all eat far too much wheat and dairy products, so these recipes will be a healthy change for everyone.

A lot of problems, I feel, come from the artificial colourings, additives, preservatives, pesticides and chemicals that are mixed with or coated onto many of today's foods. These problems can, of course, be overcome by buying organic food and washing thoroughly or peeling off all the vegetable and fruit skins. Another problem stems from chlorine in tap water. Even people who do not suffer from the most common food sensitivities may react to this, so I recommend that you use filtered or boiled water for cooking and drinking.

The nutritional value of our foods is very important, especially if you are on any restricted diet. Using this book, you will be able to construct well-balanced menus with plenty of starch, which provides sugar and fibre, to fill you up and make you feel contented. The decrease in consumption of fats will help you achieve and maintain a healthy weight, but I do advise using unsaturated fats that are unhydrogenated as this helps considerably in reducing cholesterol and heart disease. Remember it's not the bread that is fattening, but what you spread on it.

Carbohydrates are essential fillers and give you slowly released energy. You can buy very good breads such as gluten-free sourdough or corn bread, but take care to read the labels. This applies to everything we buy as, unfortunately, most foods have added wheat or yeast in them.

Cutting out dairy products means losing a lot of protein, especially in the form of cheese. Yogurt is easier to digest than milk, so some people who cannot tolerate milk may be able to eat yogurt. I often use goat's and sheep's products, as these can be tolerated by many people who are susceptible to the ill-effects of other dairy produce. In addition, they now have very sophisticated flavours and textures – quite unlike 10 years ago!

Soya is a particularly useful substitute for dairy products. Soya milk is a white liquid made exclusively from soya beans. You can buy it sweetened and with calcium, which helps to improve the taste. You can also buy soya yogurt and cream. Soya cream adds thickness and richness, but with all the optimism I possess I can't get it to whip up properly. This makes it ineffective as a filler. A more workable solution is to always have a tub of (GF/WF/DF) Swedish glacé or Tofutti ice-cream dessert that can cunningly be used to fill meringues, roulades or other puddings.

It is often the sweet finale to a meal, or particular celebrations that call for cakes and other sweet treats, that are a particular problem for those with food intolerances. For this reason, you will find a large number of desserts, cakes and sweets in this book. However, our consumption of refined sugars has increased dramatically in recent years and we need to restrict our consumption of these, so regard the wonderfully tempting sweet recipes in this book as providing you with a wide repertoire and not an excuse to eat a sumptuous dessert every night!

Don't worry if any of the ingredients in the book seem unfamiliar – they are all available at supermarkets, Italian delicatessens or health food shops. If you live some distance from a large town or city and none of these options are available or if you find it difficult to obtain the gluten, wheat and dairy-free products there are marvellous mail order companies around. You will find a helpful list of these on page 262. I have also included my list of ingredients, which might come in useful.

A professional nutritionist has assessed every recipe in this book, so you can be inspired with absolute confidence. However, do please check each recipe before you start planning, shopping or cooking, as it would be extremely annoying to find at the last minute that it is unsuited to your specific needs.

Symbols used throughout this book

The following symbols are very important. They are your guides to what is in each recipe. You can use each recipe with complete confidence knowing that a professional nutritionist has checked each recipe.

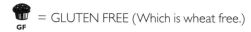 = GLUTEN FREE (Which is wheat free.)

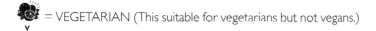 = WHEAT FREE (Which is not gluten free. However, check the recipe because you may be able to tolerate the oats or barley used.)

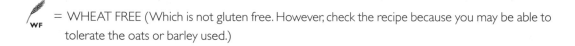 = DAIRY FREE (This is lactose free.)

= VEGETARIAN (This suitable for vegetarians but not vegans.)

= ULTRA LOW FAT (This is extremely low in fat and suitable for people on special diets.)

Any one, or all, of these symbols is printed at the top of each recipe. Please be sure that you are not allergic or intolerant to any other substances in the ingredients. Within the ingredients list in each recipe (GF), (WF) and (DF) indicates gluten free, wheat free and dairy free.

Please note that unless otherwise stated, pint measures refer to British, not American pint (20 fl oz not 16 fl oz).

Unless otherwise stated all spoon measures are level.

CHAPTER 1

Soups and Starters

Quick Seafood Soup and Rouille

A deep nostalgia for the south of France descends on me each time I make this soup. It reminds me of sun-baked terracotta, wild thyme and chilled rosé wine.

Serves 6

CHEATING ROUILLE
500ml/17fl oz/2 cups of (DF/GF) mayonnaise
1 large free-range egg yolk
A dash of (GF) French mustard and (GF) chilli sauce/oil
Salt and freshly ground black pepper

SOUP
1 large onion, peeled and finely chopped
2 tablespoons of olive oil
4 cloves of garlic, peeled and crushed
2 bay leaves
1 sprig of thyme
200g/7oz/1 cup of canned tuna fish, drained

800ml/28fl oz/3⅓ cups of carrot juice
A few drops of (GF) chilli sauce/oil
400g/14oz/2½ cups of frozen seafood cocktail, defrosted
A dash of sherry
1 tablespoon of chopped parsley, to garnish

CROÛTONS
(GF) bread
Olive oil
1 clove of garlic, peeled and crushed
Thyme
Or ready-made (GF) croûtons

First make the rouille. Mix all the ingredients in a bowl and chill until needed. Store any leftovers in a sealed jar in the refrigerator. (You can use it over the next week.)
Make the croûtons by frying small, crustless cubes of bread in olive oil, garlic and thyme. Drain on kitchen (paper) towels and keep warm.
In a large saucepan cook the onion in olive oil, until soft but not brown. Add the garlic and cook for 1 more minute. Add the herbs and then the tuna. Stir and cook for a further minute. Pour in the carrot juice and chilli sauce/oil. Leave to simmer on a medium heat for 15 minutes. Stir in the seafood and sherry and cook for 1 minute.
Remove from the heat and leave for 3 minutes.
Pour the soup into warm bowls and sprinkle with parsley. Serve with croûtons.
Transfer the rouille to a bowl and serve with the soup.

Cucumber, Coconut and Lime Soup

The transformation that fresh lime produces in any dish is instantaneous, releasing its powerful zest, and lifting the dish from the ordinary to the sublime.

Serves 10

V   GF   WF   DF

---

1 small onion, peeled and chopped

4 tablespoons of sunflower oil

2 large cucumbers, peeled, seeded and chopped

2 cloves of garlic, peeled and chopped

600ml/20fl oz/2½ cups of boiling water with 1
tablespoon of (GF) vegetable stock (bouillon)
powder

8 spring onions (scallions), trimmed and chopped

2 red chillies, seeded and chopped

2 lemon grass stalks, chopped

800ml/28fl oz/3⅓ cups of canned coconut milk

The grated rind and juice of 2 limes

Salt and freshly ground black pepper

200ml/7fl oz/¾ cup of coconut cream

2 tablespoons of chopped coriander (cilantro) leaves

Cook the onion in half the oil for 5 minutes. Add the cucumbers and garlic and gently cook for 2 minutes.

Add the water and stock (bouillon) powder. Simmer for 15 minutes; cool and liquidize.

Wash the pan and heat the remaining oil. Cook the spring onions (scallions), chillies and lemon grass over a medium heat for 2 minutes.

Stir in the cucumber liquid and add the coconut milk, grated rind and juice of 2 limes. Season to taste with salt and freshly ground black pepper.

Heat through gently for 5 minutes. Allow to cool and then chill until needed.

Stir in the coconut cream to taste, and serve in cold bowls with a sprinkling of chopped coriander (cilantro).

Winter Smoked Bacon Soup

The onset of another wet and windy day lured me to my store cupboard. With nothing more than a can of beans, I decided to conjure up a comforting soup to revive my flagging spirits.

Serves 8

1 large onion, peeled and finely chopped

1 large carrot, peeled and finely chopped

3 tablespoons of olive oil

6 thick slices of rindless smoked back bacon, chopped

4 large cloves of garlic, peeled and crushed

2 bay leaves

1.25kg/2lb 13oz/6 cups of canned butter (lima) beans (drained), or 500g/17oz/2½ cups of dried butter (lima) beans, soaked in water for 5 hours, drained and boiled for 10 minutes

1½ tablespoons of (GF) vegetable stock (bouillon) powder

2 litres/70fl oz/2 quarts of water

1 tablespoon of chopped parsley

1 tablespoon of chopped sage

Black pepper and grated nutmeg, salt if needed

A few drops of (GF) chilli sauce/oil

Cook the onion and carrot in the oil in a medium saucepan until slightly soft. Add the bacon, followed by the garlic and bay leaves and cook for 3 minutes. Stir in the beans. Pour over the water, add the stock (bouillon) powder and bring to the boil. Add half the chopped parsley and sage, plenty of seasoning and chilli sauce/oil to taste.

Reduce heat and simmer for 40 minutes. Cool slightly before liquidizing to a smooth purée. Return to the pan and reheat. Serve in warm bowls with the remaining herbs sprinkled over.

Mexican Black Bean Soup

I find black beans culinarily challenging at the best of times – their need for long hours immersed in water had discouraged me from using them, but inspired by one of the great chefs I find that they are indeed a delicacy and well worth the extra effort.

For an authentic Mexican dish serve the soup with Chilli and Herb Cornbread (see page 246).

Serves 6

1 large onion, peeled and chopped

2 red chillies, seeded and chopped

3 tablespoons of olive oil

255g/9oz/1 ½ cups of dried black beans, soaked in water overnight and then drained

1 clove of garlic, peeled and crushed

2 litres/70fl oz/2 quarts of water mixed with 2 tablespoons of (GF) vegetable stock (bouillon) powder

2 celery stalks, trimmed and sliced

2 carrots, trimmed and sliced

2 sprigs of thyme

2 bay leaves

1 teaspoon each of ground cloves and ground mace

Salt and freshly ground black pepper

3 tablespoons of chopped coriander (cilantro) leaves

In a large pan, cook the onion and chopped chillies in the oil for 5 minutes, until soft but not brown. Add the black beans and garlic. Pour in the water and stock (bouillon) powder.

Add the celery, carrots, thyme, bay leaves and spices. Season to taste and simmer for 1¹/₂ hours, or until the beans are soft. Top up with more water if necessary.

Cool, remove the bay leaves and liquidize. Adjust the seasoning if necessary.

Serve hot with a sprinkling of chopped coriander (cilantro) and slices of Chilli and Herb Cornbread.

Artichoke Soup

Artichokes are full of wonderful things that help fight off colds and generally stop you feeling under the weather. So here is a hearty and warming soup, which might help you feel good on a gloomy winter's day.

Serves 8

V   ULF   GF   WF   DF

SOUP

2 onions, peeled and thinly sliced
16 large Jerusalem artichokes, peeled and sliced
1 tablespoon of (GF) vegetable stock (bouillon)
  powder
2 litres/70fl oz/2 quarts of water
3 bay leaves
2 heaped teaspoons of mixed herbs
1 clove of garlic, peeled and crushed
1 small, mild chilli, seeded and chopped
1 tablespoon of (GF) cornflour (cornstarch)
Salt and freshly ground black pepper
400g/14oz can of artichoke hearts, drained
  and quartered

GREEN SAUCE

15g/¹/₂oz or a handful of fresh basil, with stalks
15g/¹/₂oz or a handful of fresh parsley, with stalks
15g/¹/₂oz or a handful of fresh coriander (cilantro),
  with stalks
2 tablespoons of balsamic vinegar
4 tablespoons of water
Salt and freshly ground black pepper

Place the onions, the Jerusalem artichokes and the stock (bouillon) powder in a large pan. Add the water, cover with a lid, bring to the boil and cook for 3 minutes. Drain away the water and return the onions and artichokes to the pan. Once again cover with the same amount of fresh water and, this time, add the bay leaves, herbs, garlic and chilli.

Return the pan to medium heat and bring the soup to the boil, then reduce the heat and simmer gently until all the vegetables are very soft.

Let the soup cool and then liquidize it until smooth. Place the soup back onto medium heat. Dissolve the cornflour (cornstarch) in 1 tablespoon of cold water and stir the mixture into the soup.

Bring the soup to the boil, stirring occasionally, then turn the heat down and simmer for a couple of minutes. Season to taste with salt and pepper.

Make the green sauce in a food processor. Trim the ends off the fresh herb stalks and purée the leaves and the remaining stalks with the vinegar, water and a little salt and pepper. Transfer the green sauce to a small bowl.

Stir the canned artichokes into the soup and let them get very hot. Serve the soup piping hot with a swirl of tangy green sauce in the centre.

Chilled Prawn and Cucumber Soup

In contrast to Artichoke Soup, this is a simple summer soup, refreshing and light but smart enough for entertaining. A sort of prawn (shrimp) gazpacho without the fat and calories! Please keep this soup in the refrigerator until needed, as shellfish can be so susceptible to the effects of hot sunshine.

Serves 6–8

ULF GF WF

1 ³/₄ large cucumbers, peeled and diced

400ml/14fl oz/1 ³/₄ cups of fat-free (GF) vegetable stock (bouillon) or cold water

125ml/4fl oz/¹/₂ cup of chilled tomato juice

1 red chilli, seeded and finely chopped

1 clove of garlic, peeled and crushed

500ml/17fl oz/2 cups of fat-free natural yogurt

225g/8oz/2 cups of peeled and chopped cooked prawns (shrimp), chilled

Salt and freshly ground black pepper

2 tablespoons of chopped fresh mint leaves

¹/₄ of a large cucumber kept whole for decoration

6–8 whole cooked prawns (shrimp) for decoration

Put the diced cucumber into a food processor with the stock (bouillon) or water, and process until it becomes a fine purée.

Transfer the mixture to a large serving bowl and stir in the tomato juice, chilli and garlic. Mix in the yogurt, chopped prawns (shrimp), salt and pepper, chopped mint and taste it!

Cover the soup with clingfilm (plastic wrap) and chill for a couple of hours to allow the flavours to develop.

Decorate the chilled soup before serving. First, wipe clean the skin of the remaining cucumber quarter, then cut it into 12–16 thin slices. Place two overlapping slices of cucumber in the centre of the soup and place one of the reserved prawns (shrimp) on top.

Pickled Ginger, Lemon Grass and Mussel Soup

The impact of pickled ginger is balanced by the subtleties of fresh lemon grass. I keep both in the refrigerator for stir-fries and curries.

Serves 6

ULF   GF   WF   DF

1 tablespoon of sesame oil	600ml/20fl oz/2 ½ cups of water
6 spring onions (scallions), trimmed and chopped	140g/5oz of pickled ginger slices, drained
1 red chilli, seeded and chopped	1 teaspoon of (GF) fish sauce (or double up on [GF]
2 cloves of garlic, peeled and crushed	soy sauce)
2 stalks of lemon grass, finely sliced	1 teaspoon of dark (GF) soy sauce
1kg/2.2lb of prepared fresh (or frozen) mussels in or	Salt and freshly ground black pepper
out of shells	1 bunch of fresh coriander (cilantro), chopped
425g/15oz of condensed beef consommé	

Heat the oil in a large pan. Add the onions (scallions), chilli, garlic and lemon grass.
Cook for 3 minutes.
Add the mussels, followed by the consommé, water, pickled ginger, fish sauce and soy sauce.
Season and then simmer for 10 minutes.
Serve the soup immediately in hot bowls and sprinkle with the chopped coriander (cilantro).

Clam Soup

Now that I have discovered some decent canned clams, I am converted into a clam chowder fan! This particularly light version of the all-American soup is made with fresh clams and tuna so that it is complete low-fat meal in itself. Serve with fresh, warm bread.

Serves 6

1 large onion, peeled and very finely chopped
1 litre/35fl oz/4 cups of water
1 litre/35fl oz/4 cups of (GF) fish stock (bouillon)
2 cloves of garlic, peeled and crushed
2 bay leaves
1 sprig of fresh thyme

140ml/5fl oz/^{2}/₃ cup of good white wine (Burgundy is perfect)
200g/7oz/1 cup of tuna fish in brine or water, drained
A few drops of (GF) chilli sauce/oil
1kg/2.2lbs/4 cups of fresh clams (shells on)
6 large sprigs of fresh parsley, finely chopped

Put the onion and water into a large pan over high heat, cover with a lid and bring it to the boil. Cook for 5 minutes and then drain away the water. Put the onions back into the pan and once again cover them with the same amount of fresh water. This time add the stock (bouillon) as well and cook over medium heat for about 10 minutes.

Add the garlic, bay leaves, thyme and wine and simmer for another 10 minutes. Reduce the heat and simmer until the onions are soft and the liquid has reduced by about half.

Mix in the tuna fish, chilli sauce/oil, clams and half the parsley and simmer gently until the clams are heated through. Do not boil the soup or the clams will become rubbery. Serve the soup immediately with the remaining fresh parsley sprinkled over.

Tomato Mousse and Avocado Ceviche

Here, the traditional Mexican mix of tomatoes, avocados, black beans, coriander (cilantro) and limes are put together in a more European way as an ideal starter.

Serves 6

100g/3½oz/½ cup of dried black beans, soaked
   in water overnight
2 ripe avocados, skinned, stoned (pitted)
   and chopped
2 beef tomatoes, skinned, seeded and chopped
1 red chilli, seeded and chopped
1 small red onion, peeled and very finely chopped
The juice of 3 limes, and grated rind of 2 of them
Salt and freshly ground black pepper
2 tablespoons of olive oil
3 tablespoons of coconut cream
1 teaspoon of coriander (cilantro) seeds, crushed
Large bunch of coriander (cilantro) leaves

MOUSSE
Sunflower oil for greasing
700g/24oz/3 cups of tomato passata
(GF) chilli sauce/oil and (GF) Worcestershire sauce
The juice of ½ a lemon
11.7g/½oz sachet (US 1 tablespoon) of powdered
   gelatine or vegetarian equivalent
40g/1½oz of rocket (arugula) leaves, washed and
   dried

6 ramekins, greased with sunflower oil and lined
   with baking parchment (wax paper)

The day before you need them, cook the soaked beans in boiling water until soft.
To make the ceviche, first drain and then mix the beans in a large bowl with the avocado, tomatoes, chilli, onion, lime juice and zest, seasoning, olive oil, coconut cream, coriander (cilantro) seeds and half of the chopped coriander (cilantro) leaves.
Marinate overnight or for at least 4 hours, stirring occasionally.
To make the mousse, mix the tomato passata with the chilli and Worcestershire sauce, lemon juice and seasoning to taste.
Dissolve the gelatine by stirring it into about 2 tablespoons of boiling water in a cup until it is clear and there are no lumps.
Stir this into the tomato mixture and place in the refrigerator to chill and thicken slightly.
After about 10 minutes, spoon the mousse into each ramekin and level off. Chill until set.
Cut the rocket (arugula) stems in half, and arrange on each plate.
Turn out each mousse onto the plate by briefly dipping the ramekins into a bowl of boiling water.
Remove the paper, spoon the avocado ceviche around the mousse.
Serve with Sesame Corn Crackers (*see page 250*), or Chilli and Herb Cornbread (*see page 246*).

Rocket, Fennel and Strawberry Salad

Always eat fresh strawberries at room temperature, as they lose their delicate flavour and natural sweetness when chilled. For sheer extravagance and a romantic dinner for two, you could use fraises de bois – *cultivated 'wild' strawberries which are only available at exclusive stores.*

Serves 4

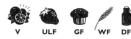

100g/3½oz/4 large handfuls of fresh, ready-to-eat baby rocket (arugula) leaves

1 large bulb of fresh fennel, trimmed and tough outer layers removed

300g/10½oz/2 heaped cups of fresh strawberries, wiped clean and hulled

1 teaspoon of crushed coriander (cilantro) seeds

1 teaspoon of mild (GF) Dijon mustard

1 tablespoon of red wine vinegar

1 small mild red chilli, seeded and finely chopped

The juice of 1 large sweet orange

Arrange the rocket (arugula) leaves on each plate.

Using a very sharp knife, cut the fennel in half and then into wafer thin slices. Divide the fennel slices between the salads.

Cut the strawberries into thick slices and arrange them over the salads. (If you do succumb to the temptation of *fraises de bois* then keep the strawberries whole.)

Make the dressing in a small bowl by mixing together the coriander (cilantro) seeds, mustard, vinegar, chilli and orange juice. Whisk the dressing until it is smooth, drizzle it over the salads and serve.

Potato Skins and Hummus Dip

An almost instantaneous starter at any time of the year. Brilliant for barbecues, hungry teenagers and vegetarians. Use ready-made wafers (chips) (GF/WF/DF) if you are in a real hurry!

Serves 8

Home-made fried potato skin quarters, or 500g/17oz of (GF/DF) ready-made fried potato skins, or 200g/7oz of (WF/GF) ready-made wafers (chips)

Salt and freshly ground black pepper

840g/30oz/4 cups of canned chickpeas (garbanzo beans), drained

2 tablespoons of light tahini paste

3 large cloves of garlic, peeled and chopped

A few drops of (GF) chilli sauce/oil

The juice of 2 large lemons

297g/10½oz of silken tofu (firm)

At least 3 tablespoons of fresh coriander (cilantro) leaves

Cayenne pepper

A little chopped parsley for decoration

Preheat the oven to 200°C/400°F/Gas mark 6

Place the potato skins on a non-stick baking sheet and sprinkle with salt and pepper. Bake in the preheated oven until crispy.

Meanwhile, mix the chickpeas (garbanzo beans), tahini, garlic, chilli sauce/oil, lemon juice, tofu, salt, pepper and coriander (cilantro)

leaves together in the food processor until smooth.

Scoop into an attractive bowl. Sprinkle with cayenne pepper and parsley.

Place in the centre of a large oval plate and arrange the potato skins around the dip.

Serve immediately.

Roast Artichoke, Fennel and Onion Salad

Once laborious to peel, Jerusalem artichokes have now been perfected into a less complex shape. I have now been converted to these underrated vegetables as an alternative to potatoes.

Serves 4

V   GF   WF   DF

500g/17oz of fresh Jerusalem artichokes (washed, peeled and left in a bowl of cold water and a teaspoon of fresh lemon juice to prevent discolouration)

(GF) chilli oil and olive oil

2 heads of fennel, trimmed and quartered

2 large onions, peeled and quartered

Salt and freshly ground black pepper

2 cloves of garlic, peeled and crushed

Fresh marjoram

The juice of 1 lemon

Preheat the oven to 200°C/400°F/Gas mark 6

Cook the artichokes in boiling water for 10 minutes. Drain and rinse under cold water. Sprinkle a large non-stick baking sheet with the oils. Mix the vegetables together and spread over the sheet. Sprinkle with more of the oils, salt and pepper, crushed garlic and the marjoram. Place the tray in the centre of the oven and roast until golden, about ³/₄–1 hour.
Carefully spoon the vegetables into a salad bowl and sprinkle with the lemon juice. Serve with warm (GF) bread, or cover and chill until needed.

Prawn and Pepper Terrine

This terrine is bright and colourful, so there is no need to feel gloomy if you have to give a low-fat dinner party! If you entertain a lot, you can substitute other low-fat seafood or fish, and the peppers can be swapped for any suitable and complementary vegetables. You can also use a ring mould instead of a terrine tin and fill the centre with the salad leaves.

Serves 8

ULF   GF WF DF

2 x 22g/³/₄oz sachets of (GF) aspic jelly powder
900ml/32fl oz/4 scant cups of boiling water
100ml/3¹/₂fl oz/scant ¹/₂ cup of dry sherry
Salt and freshly ground black pepper
A few drops of (GF) chilli sauce/oil
55–85g/2–3oz/1 cup dwarf French green beans, trimmed and cut into thirds
1 yellow pepper, cored and seeded

A small bunch of fresh coriander (cilantro) leaves
400g/14oz/2 generous cups of fresh, large peeled prawns (shrimp)
3 ripe tomatoes, skinned, seeded and cut into eighths
Rocket (arugula) and watercress leaves
Fresh lemon juice
30.5cm/12 inch terrine tin or a standard size non-stick ring mould

Dissolve both the sachets of aspic jelly powder in a large jug with the boiling water. Add the sherry, seasoning and chilli sauce/oil to taste. Leave the jelly to cool and then transfer it to the refrigerator so that it can thicken up a little. Keep watching the jelly so that it does not become too thick to handle.

Meanwhile, blanch the green beans in boiling water for 3 minutes, drain and refresh under cold water. Cut the pepper into bite size pieces. Choose some of the best coriander (cilantro) leaves and set the rest aside to mix in with your salad garnish. Arrange rows of prawns (shrimps), green beans, yellow pepper, coriander (cilantro) leaves and tomatoes all the way across and down the length of the terrine tin in any design you like.

Spoon the slightly thickened, cold aspic jelly all over the design until you have a thin, smooth layer covering the seafood and vegetables. Put it in the deep freeze for a few minutes until set. Repeat this in continuous layers until all the ingredients and jelly are used up.

Cover the terrine with clingfilm (plastic wrap) and chill until completely firm and set. I suggest at least 4 more hours.

Uncover the terrine. Dip the base of the tin into a basin of boiling water for a second then, using a sharp knife, ease the jelly from around the edges of the tin and quickly turn it onto the centre of an oblong serving dish.

Mix the rocket (arugula) leaves, watercress and reserved coriander (cilantro). Toss the leaves in a little lemon juice and black pepper (or some really good fat-free salad dressing). Arrange the salad around the base of the terrine and serve immediately, or keep it in the refrigerator until needed.

Spinach and Cheese Moulds

For special occasions, you can add a few chopped prawns (shrimp) to the cheese filling and then decorate the moulds with whole prawns (shrimp) on a bed of salad leaves. I often change the filling to include pieces of chopped mild red chilli and red pepper.

Serves 4–6

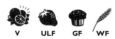

CHEESE MOULDS

170g/6oz/3 cups of fresh, young spinach leaves, trimmed

500g/17oz/2 generous cups of virtually fat-free fromage frais

1 small clove of garlic, peeled and crushed

200g/7oz/1¼ cups of cooked and drained sweetcorn kernels

2 heaped tablespoons of shredded fresh basil leaves

Salt and freshly ground black pepper

A little freshly grated nutmeg

11.7g/½oz sachet (US 1 tablespoon) powdered gelatine or vegetarian equivalent, dissolved according to the instructions on the packet

TOMATO AND RED PEPPER SAUCE

1 teaspoon of cumin powder

400g/14oz/2 cups of canned plum tomatoes in natural juice

400g/14oz/2 cups of canned pimentos (sweet peppers) in natural juice, drained

A few drops of (GF) chilli sauce/oil

Salt and freshly ground black pepper

4–6 ramekins or tin moulds, lined on the base with a circle of baking parchment (wax paper)

Fresh basil leaves or whole baby sweetcorn and fresh rocket (arugula) leaves to decorate

Cook the spinach in a saucepan with a little water until just wilted. Do not over-cook it, 3 minutes should be enough. Drain the spinach and pat it dry with kitchen (paper) towels. Make the sauce. Purée the cumin with the tomatoes and pimentos in a food processor. Add the chilli sauce/oil according to taste and season with salt and pepper. Transfer the sauce to a jug and chill in the refrigerator until needed.

Line the ramekins or moulds with the spinach leaves, covering the base and letting the leaves overhang the edges enough to enable you to fold them back into the middle.

Mix the fromage frais with the garlic, sweetcorn, basil, salt, pepper and nutmeg in a bowl. Stir in the dissolved gelatine, then spoon the mixture into each ramekin and smooth over. Now gently pull the spinach leaves over the filling and cover it with more leaves, if necessary, so that there is no filling showing.

Place in the refrigerator for at least 4 hours to set.

Loosen the edges of the spinach away from its mould and turn each one out onto the centre of a serving plate. Remove the circle of paper and drizzle the tomato and red pepper sauce over the moulds.

Decorate around the moulds with fresh basil leaves or, for special occasions, place a star of halved baby sweetcorn around each one and serve on a bed of rocket (arugula). Serve chilled.

Pumpkin and Cheese Tart

Pumpkins are now widely available and are just as popular in England as in the USA. Here is an interesting and unusual recipe for you to try.

Serves 6

PASTRY
100g/3½oz/²/₃ cup of brown rice flour
70g/2½oz/½ cup of maize flour
70g/2½oz/½ cup of porridge oats
½ teaspoon of salt
115g/4oz/½ cup of (DF) margarine
1 large free-range egg, beaten
1 tablespoon of olive oil

FILLING
600g/21oz of pumpkin flesh, peeled and seeded
4 tablespoons of olive oil
1 small onion, peeled and sliced

1 teaspoon of fresh thyme leaves
1 clove of garlic, peeled and crushed
Salt and freshly ground black pepper
Grated nutmeg
130g/4½oz/²/₃ cup of grated goat's or sheep's
   cheese, or vegetarian cheese
240ml/8fl oz/1 cup of goat's or sheep's yogurt
3 large free-range eggs, beaten
A pinch of cayenne pepper and a bunch of lamb's
   lettuce (mâche)

24cm/10 inch non-stick, loose-bottomed, fluted
   flan tin

Preheat the oven to 200°C/400°F/Gas mark 6

Place the flours, oats, salt and margarine in a food processor and mix for a second or two until it resembles fine breadcrumbs. Mix the egg and oil together and pour into the food processor with the machine running. Turn out the mixture onto a floured board and, with floured hands, bring into a ball of dough. Wrap in clingfilm (plastic wrap)and chill for 30 minutes.
Roll out on a floured board and line the flan tin. Prick the bottom with a fork and chill for 1 hour. Line the pastry with greaseproof (wax) paper and ceramic beans and bake for 10 minutes. Remove the balls and paper and bake for a further 25 minutes. Cool until needed. Turn down the oven to 180°C/350°F/Gas mark 4.
Cut the pumpkin into thin wedges and blanch in boiling water for 5 minutes until softened. Heat half the oil and fry the pumpkin slices for 10 minutes to brown them on each side. Drain on kitchen (paper) towels. Add the remaining oil and cook the onion with the thyme and garlic, until soft, but not brown. Season with salt, pepper and grated nutmeg and cover the pastry base with the mixture. Arrange the pumpkin wedges on top and all around the flan.
Mix the cheese, yogurt and eggs together with a little more seasoning and spoon over evenly. Sprinkle with a little cayenne pepper and bake for 45 minutes, or until puffy and firm and the pumpkin is cooked through.
Serve warm, or cold, with lamb's lettuce (mâche), drizzled with virgin olive oil and black pepper.

Sweet Pepper Tart

Grilling (broiling) the peppers is crucial to bring out the intense sweet flavour vital to the success of this tart. The skins should blister with black spots before being peeled off.

Serves 6

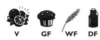

4 large red peppers, cored and seeded

Olive oil

1 plump clove of garlic, peeled and crushed

1 teaspoon of marjoram leaves

1 teaspoon of balsamic vinegar

240ml/8fl oz/1 cup of soya cream

6 large free-range egg yolks

Salt and freshly ground black pepper

A little caster (superfine) sugar

A few drops of (GF) chilli sauce/oil

Pre-baked (WF/DF) shortcrust pastry case made in a 24cm/10 inch non-stick, loose-bottomed fluted flan tin (see *page 16*)

Cayenne pepper

140g/5oz of lamb's lettuce (mâche)

Preheat the oven to 200°C/400°F/Gas mark 6

Brush the peppers with olive oil and grill (broil) until charred and blistered. Leave to cool and then peel off the skin with a sharp knife and discard. Chop up the peppers, then cook them in a tablespoon of oil with the garlic and marjoram for 2 minutes. Add the balsamic vinegar to the pan and cook for 3 minutes. Set aside to cool a little.

Put the cream, eggs and cooled peppers in a food processor and blend until smooth. Adjust the seasoning with salt, pepper, sugar and chilli sauce/oil and blend again. Scrape the mixture into the prepared pastry case. Sprinkle lightly with cayenne pepper and bake for 25–30 minutes or until set.

Cut into wedges and serve warm with a little lamb's lettuce (mâche) sprinkled with olive oil and black pepper around each piece.

Pink Grapefruit and Ginger Salad

Without doubt the easiest and quickest recipe in the book. Ideal for reluctant hosts or hectic hostesses. Ordinary grapefruits are too acidic as a starter, so the pinker the better.

Serves 8

255g/9oz of parsley, trimmed and chopped
Salt and freshly ground black pepper
2 plump cloves of garlic, peeled and crushed
1 teaspoon of balsamic vinegar

6 tablespoons of olive oil
10cm/4 inch of root ginger, peeled
6 large pink/red grapefruit, peeled
40g/1½oz of lamb's lettuce (mâche)

Make the dressing in a large bowl by beating together three quarters of the chopped parsley with seasoning, garlic, vinegar and oil. Grate in all of the ginger. Segment the grapefruit, removing all the pith, skin and pips (seeds) and marinate in the dressing until needed (up to 24 hours). Keep covered in the refrigerator.

Serve on plates with lamb's lettuce (mâche) and crispy warm (GF) bread.

Smoked Mackerel Pâté

This recipe transforms boring old tofu into a delicious pâté. In 55g/2oz of tofu there are 300mg of calcium so it is an excellent alternative to the cheese products we'd normally use.

Serves 6

GF WF DF

4 fillets of smoked mackerel, skinned
297g/10¹/₂oz of silken tofu (firm)
The juice of ¹/₂ a lemon
1 teaspoon of (GF/DF) hot horseradish relish or
  a few drops of (GF) chilli sauce/oil

Salt and freshly ground black pepper
Cayenne pepper
Slices of (GF) bread or pure maize corn chips

Put the mackerel, tofu, lemon juice, horseradish or chilli sauce/oil, salt and freshly ground black pepper into the food processor and process until just smooth.
Spoon into a serving dish. Sprinkle with cayenne pepper and serve with toasted slices of (GF) bread or corn chips, or cover and chill until needed.

Wild Rice and Smoked Trout Blinis

I found it mildly surprising that this recipe actually worked! Its nutty flavour is well matched by the subtleties of smoked trout. This dish is delicious with chilled vodka and will certainly get the party going.

Serves 6 (2 each)

DRESSING

2 tablespoons of capers, drained

55g/2oz/½ cup of anchovies, drained and finely chopped

The juice and rind of 1 large lemon

4 tablespoons of olive oil

Salt and freshly ground black pepper

1 sprig of fresh rosemary leaves, very finely chopped

1 teaspoon of honey

4 whole Arbroath smokies/smoked trout

BLINIS

70g/2½oz/½ cup of well-cooked wild rice

170g/6oz/1 cup plus 3 tablespoons of buckwheat flour

1 large free-range egg

300ml/10fl oz/1¼ cups of sheep's or goat's yogurt

1 teaspoon salt

1 teaspoon of (GF) baking powder

2 tablespoons of sunflower oil (and some more for frying)

½ teaspoon of bicarbonate of soda (baking soda)

1 tablespoon of boiling water

500g/17oz/2 cups of Greek set sheep's yogurt

2 tablespoons of chopped parsley

Freshly ground black pepper

Make the dressing first by whisking all of the ingredients in a bowl. Cover and chill in the refrigerator until needed.

Remove all the skin and bones from the Arbroath smokies and break into attractive pieces. Cover and chill.

Next make the blinis. In a food processor briefly beat the flour, egg, yogurt, salt, baking powder and oil into a smooth batter. Mix this gently into the rice. Dissolve the bicarbonate of soda (baking soda) with the hot water and stir quickly into the mixture.

Cover the base of a frying pan (skillet) with oil. Heat the oil until it is hot enough to fry a tablespoon of batter until it sizzles and becomes golden and puffy. Flip the blini over and cook on the other side until golden. Make 12 blinis.

Keep them warm on a dish covered with a clean damp tea towel. Use more oil as necessary.

Place a warm blini on each plate. Pile on the smoked trout. Spoon over a blob of yogurt, sprinkle with parsley and black pepper.

Drizzle the dressing around the blinis and serve immediately.

Warm Scallops and Fennel with Tomato Dill Dressing

Dynamic yet simple is how I prefer my scallops. Briefly cooked so that they still impart the flavour of the ocean – never stewed or frazzled.

Serves 4

GF WF DF

4 bulbs of fennel, trimmed and quartered

Extra virgin olive oil for brushing and serving

1/2 red onion, peeled and finely chopped

1 tablespoon of olive oil

1 tablespoon of (DF) margarine

4 tablespoons of white wine

455g/16oz/4 cups of fresh or frozen, defrosted scallops (without coral)

4 tablespoons of tomato passata

15g/1/2oz/1/2 cup of fresh dill, chopped

Salt and freshly ground black pepper

4 scallop shells, cleaned

Preheat the oven to 200°C/400°F/Gas mark 6

Brush the fennel with oil and bake in the oven until browned and the edges have softened, about 45 minutes.

Cook the onion in the oil and margarine until soft.

Add the wine, cook for another minute and then add the scallops. Cook for a further minute, turning once.

Add the tomato passata, dill, salt and pepper, and continue to cook for 1 more minute.

Spoon the mixture into the shells and serve in the centre of large warm plates surrounded by the fennel quarters.

Drizzle with any remaining sauce and a little extra virgin olive oil, then sprinkle with black pepper.

Crab Mousse with Pear Vinaigrette

The craze for pink peppercorns is no longer with us. Now, of course, they are easily purchased in any reputable supermarket and we no longer have to scour the shelves of smart delicatessens.

Serves 6

GF / WF / DF

11.7g/¹/₂oz sachet (US 1 tablespoon) of powdered gelatine

2 dressed crabs, fresh or frozen and defrosted

2 tablespoons of (DF/GF) mayonnaise

(GF) chilli sauce/oil to taste

(GF) Worcestershire sauce to taste

The juice of ¹/₂ a lemon

Salt and freshly ground black pepper

2 tablespoons of soya cream

1 egg white, stiffly beaten

410g/14¹/₂oz/2 cups of pear quarters in natural juices

2 tablespoons of olive oil

The juice of 2 limes

2 teaspoons of pink peppercorns, drained

6 ramekins or moulds, lined on the base with a circle of baking parchment (wax paper)

Dissolve the gelatine in 3 tablespoons of boiling water and stir until it is clear and lump-free. In a bowl, mix the crab meat, mayonnaise, sauces, lemon juice and seasoning with the cream. Stir in the gelatine, fold in the egg white and spoon the mousse into each mould. Cover with clingfilm (plastic wrap) and chill for 3–4 hours.

When ready to serve, drain the pears and slice them.

Dip the ramekins or moulds into a little boiling water to loosen, then turn them out onto plates. Remove the baking parchment (wax paper). Arrange the pear slices around each mousse.

Mix the oil, lime juice and peppercorns with salt and pepper, and drizzle over the pears.

Smoked Salmon Turbans

Smoked salmon and the Christmas festivities seem unequivocally bound together. Unmistakably luxurious, salmon is a special treat meriting little or no alteration from its natural state. However, this recipe does help a little go a long way.

Serves 8

GF WF DF

11.7g/½oz sachet (US 1 tablespoon) of powdered gelatine

550g/19oz of salmon fillet, all bones and skin removed

A few slices of lemon

Salt and freshly ground black pepper

297g/10½oz of tofu (set firm)

1 teaspoon of tomato purée (paste)

2 tablespoons of lemon juice

A few drops of (GF) Tabasco sauce/chilli oil

3 teaspoons of dry sherry

455g/16oz of sliced smoked salmon

2 packets of watercress, trimmed

Extra virgin olive oil

2 large lemons, cut into 8 wedges

8 ramekins or moulds, lined with clingfilm (plastic wrap)

Dissolve the gelatine in 3 tablespoons of boiling water and stir until it is clear and lump-free. Meanwhile, wrap the salmon in foil with a little water, a few slices of lemon, salt and pepper. Poach for 15 minutes.

Open the foil and leave to cool. Flake the fish into a bowl, add the juices and then briefly process the tofu, fish and juices in a food processor with the tomato, lemon juice and Tabasco. Stir in the gelatine and beat thoroughly until pink, creamy and smooth.

Transfer to a bowl and fold in the sherry using a metal spoon. Line each ramekin or mould with clingfilm (plastic wrap), then line the clingfilm (plastic wrap) with salmon slices, making sure that there are no holes and that there is an overlap to fold over to encase the mousse.

Divide the mousse between the ramekins, then smooth over and seal up with the overlapping salmon. Cover with clingfilm (plastic wrap) and chill for 4 hours or more. Turn out onto the centre of each plate, surround with watercress and drizzle with the oil and pepper.

Serve each turban with a wedge of lemon and a plate of thinly sliced Cumin Seed and Rye Bread (not GF) (*see page 244*) or (GF) bread of your choice.

Avocado and Fresh Salmon Corn Meal Pancakes

These pancakes are ideal for breakfast with bacon and eggs on top, or scrambled eggs and smoked salmon for special occasions. They are also superb with avocado and bacon, fresh prawns or crab as a starter or even a light lunch.

Serves 6

455g/16oz of fresh skinless and boneless salmon fillet
   cut into 2cm/³/4 inch cubes
240ml/8fl oz/1 cup of fresh lime juice
2 chillies, seeded and finely chopped
Salt and freshly ground black pepper
2 ripe avocado pears, peeled and stoned (pitted)
1 very large tomato, skinned and finely chopped

CORN MEAL PANCAKES
115g/4oz/³/4 cup of sifted fine corn meal
115g/4oz/³/4 cup of sifted white rice flour
3 heaped teaspoons of (GF) baking powder
1 teaspoon of salt
Freshly ground black pepper
2 eggs, lightly beaten
240ml/8fl oz/1 cup of goat's yogurt

Oil for frying
3 tablespoons of chopped fresh coriander
   (cilantro) leaves

Start 2–24 hours before eating. In a china or glass bowl, marinate the fish in the lime juice with the chillies and seasoning until it is opaque. Keep chilled and cover with clingfilm (plastic wrap).

When you are ready to make the pancakes, chop up the avocados into cubes and add to the lime juice with the tomato.

Just before serving, make the pancakes. Mix the dry ingredients together in one bowl and the liquid ingredients in another, then quickly but thoroughly stir them together.

Heat a little oil in a non-stick frying pan (skillet) and make 6 pancakes, using about 3 spoonfuls of batter for each one.

Cook over a medium heat for 3–4 minutes, turning once, until cooked right through and golden on both sides.

Keep the pancakes warm in a low oven until they are all prepared.

To serve, place each pancake on a hot plate. Drain the salmon and avocado mixture and arrange the topping over the pancakes. Sprinkle with the coriander (cilantro) and serve at once.

Beetroot Jellies with Celeriac Remoulade

Celeriac remoulade is used rather like a jumped-up coleslaw. Usually it is made with lashing of olive oil and far more vinegar and mustard than would ordinarily be used in any mayonnaise. This recipe however, being a fat-free version, has no oil at all.

Serves 6

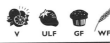

BEETROOT (BEET) JELLIES

1 bunch small spring onions (scallions), trimmed and sliced
1 teaspoon of cumin powder
Salt and freshly ground black pepper
140ml/5fl oz/²/₃ cup of water
140ml/5fl oz/²/₃ cup of dry white wine
12 small or 8 medium, whole pre-cooked beetroots (beets), trimmed, peeled and chopped
A few drops of (GF) chilli sauce/oil
1¹/₂ sachets (16g/³/₄oz/US 1¹/₂ tablespoons) of powdered gelatine, dissolved according to the instructions on the packet, or vegetarian equivalent

CELERIAC REMOULADE

425g/15oz/5 cups of fresh, shredded celeriac
Salt and freshly ground black pepper
Juice of ¹/₂ a lemon
3 tablespoons of (GF) Dijon mustard
2–3 tablespoons of boiling water
1 tablespoon of wine vinegar
4 heaped tablespoons of virtually fat-free fromage frais
2 heaped tablespoons of chopped fresh parsley

Some fresh herbs to decorate
6 ramekins or tin moulds, lined on the base with a circle of baking parchment (wax paper)

Place the spring onions (scallions), cumin powder, salt, pepper, water and wine in a non-stick saucepan and gently cook over medium heat until the onions are nearly soft. Add the beetroot (beets) to the pan, heat through and season to taste with chilli sauce/oil. Set aside for 20 minutes. When cool, purée the mixture in a food processor. With the machine still running, add the dissolved gelatine to the purée so that it is evenly distributed.

Fill each of the prepared ramekins or moulds with the purée, cover with clingfilm (plastic wrap) and chill in the refrigerator for at least 4 hours or until set

Meanwhile, place the celeriac in a bowl with the remaining remoulade ingredients and mix gently. The sauce should be firm enough to spoon the celeriac into a pile without the sauce running all over the plate! Adjust the seasoning to taste, cover with clingfilm (plastic wrap) and chill for at least 2 hours or until needed.

Dip the bottom of the moulds into hot water and then loosen the jellies using a sharp knife. Remove the circles of paper. Place a spoonful of the celeriac remoulade beside each jelly and decorate with a few fresh herbs. Serve immediately, or chill until needed.

CHAPTER 2

Vegetable Dishes

Stir-fry Cabbage and Ginger

Humble Savoy cabbage is transformed in seconds into a delectable but simple accompaniment to roasted or grilled (broiled) meats, game or poultry.

Serves 6–8

V   GF   WF   DF

1 large Savoy cabbage

3 tablespoons of sunflower oil

2 tablespoons of mild (GF) chilli oil

8cm/3 inch root ginger, peeled and grated

Salt and freshly ground black pepper

1 tablespoon of (DF) margarine, or (GF) chilli oil
  for serving

Halve the cabbage, remove any hard white core/stem and slice very finely.

Heat the oils in a wok and fry the cabbage with the ginger, salt and pepper until just softened.

Serve hot with the margarine or chilli oil dotted all over it, and a little black pepper.

Exotic Pea Purée

An exotic version of the popular English dish, mushy peas, this is delicious with roast or grilled (broiled) fish, meat and poultry and its vivid colour brightens up the simplest lamb chop.

Serves 6–8

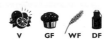

1kg/2.2lb/8 cups of frozen peas
1 large bunch of coriander (cilantro) or 3 × 15g/½oz supermarket packets
Salt and freshly ground black pepper to taste

Grated nutmeg to taste
Dash of (GF) chilli sauce/oil
1 tablespoon (DF) margarine
200ml/7fl oz/¾ cup of coconut cream

Cook the peas in salted boiling water until tender, about 3–5 minutes. Drain and process half of them in a food processor. Scrape the mixture into a bowl.

Remove the stalks from the coriander (cilantro) and discard them. (The supermarket packets are usually trimmed.)

Place the rest of the peas with the coriander (cilantro) leaves and remaining ingredients in the food processor and process until smooth. Scrape this mixture into the first pea purée and blend together. Adjust the seasoning to taste. Transfer to a warm serving dish and cover until needed.

Nutty Vegetable Roulade

This enticing vegetarian dish is ideal for Christmas lunch. You can also change the filling from sweetcorn into a non-vegetarian left-over turkey recipe after Christmas.

Serves 6

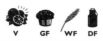

FILLING
340g/12oz of parsnips, peeled and chopped
30g/1oz/2 tablespoons of (DF) margarine
2 tablespoons of soya cream
Freshly grated nutmeg
455g/16oz/2 1/3 cups of whole sweetcorn, drained

1 teaspoon of fresh thyme leaves
Salt and freshly ground black pepper
130g/4 1/2 oz/1 cup of grated courgette (zucchini)
100g/3 1/2 oz/3/4 cup of chopped, toasted mixed nuts
3 large free-range eggs, separated
Cayenne pepper

ROULADE
40g/1 1/2 oz/3 tablespoons of (DF) margarine
30g/1oz/scant 1/4 cup of rice flour
300ml/10fl oz/1 1/4 cups of unsweetened soya milk

A large non-stick roulade tin, greased with (DF)
    margarine and lined with baking parchment
    (wax paper)

Preheat the oven to 200°C/400°F/Gas mark 6

Boil the parsnips until soft. Drain and then mash them with the margarine, soya cream and nutmeg until smooth. Season to taste with salt and pepper. Stir in the sweetcorn, cover and keep warm.

Make the roulade by first melting the margarine. Beat in the flour and then incorporate the milk until you have a smooth sauce. Season to taste with thyme, salt and pepper. Stir in the grated courgette (zucchini), half the mixed nuts and the egg yolks and remove from the heat.

In a large bowl, whisk the egg whites until stiff, then spoon one tablespoonful into the courgette (zucchini) mixture and blend gently. Now fold in the remaining egg whites very carefully using a metal spoon.

Scrape the mixture into the prepared tin and sprinkle with a little cayenne pepper.

Bake for 15–20 minutes until puffy but firm. Turn the roulade onto a piece of baking parchment (wax paper) that has been sprinkled with the remaining nuts.

Peel off the baking paper. Slice off the ends if they look a little dry. Spread the warm filling mixture over the roulade and gently use the paper underneath to help you roll up the roulade.

Slide the roulade carefully onto a warm serving dish and decorate with fresh parsley. Accompany the dish with Cranberry Sauce (*see page 83*).

Wild Mushrooms with Lentils Provençal

*Autumn walks in the woods, with glorious coloured leaves and crisp, clean air is to me one of
the marvels of nature. Nestling under the leaves and around the huge old trees bloom delicious wild
mushrooms to be collected along the way.*
This lovely French recipe can be used with fresh or dried mushrooms of your choice.

Serves 4

V   ULF   GF   WF   DF

1 litre/35fl oz/4 cups of water
1 large red onion, peeled and thinly sliced
255g/9oz/1½ cups of Puy or green lentils
240ml/8fl oz/1 cup of sweet red vermouth
1 tablespoon of (GF) vegetable stock
   (bouillon) powder

Salt and freshly ground black pepper
Freshly grated nutmeg
3 sprigs of fresh rosemary
40g/1½oz/2 cups of dried, mixed wild mushrooms
   (any quantity of fresh ones)

Boil the water in a non-stick pan, add the onion and cook for about 10 minutes. Add the lentils
and continue cooking over medium–high heat for another 10 minutes, stirring from time to time.
(If the liquid reduces too much, add some more water.)

Pour in the vermouth and cook for 5 minutes. Now stir in the stock (bouillon) powder, salt and
pepper, nutmeg and rosemary, reduce the heat and simmer for 15 minutes.

Finally, mix in the mushrooms and leave the pot to simmer for about 20 minutes. Adjust the
seasoning and serve with warm bread and a fresh green salad.

Honey Glazed Turnips

It's virtually impossible to get me to eat a turnip, but seduced by the idea of wild honey and thyme I succumbed to bribery. I now treat them with respectful awe, amazed that anything so bland can be transformed into something so delicious.

Serves 6–8

---

24 baby turnips, peeled and trimmed

2 heaped tablespoons of (GF/DF) four-grain mustard

6 tablespoons of wild runny honey

2 tablespoons of sunflower oil

Salt and freshly ground black pepper

2 heaped teaspoons of fresh thyme leaves

Preheat the oven to 180°C/350°F/Gas mark 4

Add the turnips to a pan of boiling water. Return to the boil and cook for 5 minutes just to soften them. Drain and refresh under hot water and leave to dry out a bit.

Gently heat the mustard, honey and oil together and season with a little salt and pepper.

Place the turnips on a non-stick baking sheet, pour the honey over them and sprinkle with thyme. Bake in the oven until golden brown and sticky, about 1 3/4 hours, or until cooked through, basting occasionally with the glaze so that they brown evenly.

Celeriac Dauphinoise

You can always replace half of the celeriac with potato slices if you find this recipe too expensive. It has a soft and delicious flavour and is ideal with grilled (broiled) fish, game and roasts of all sorts.

Serves 8

2 celeriac roots, peeled, quartered and very
   thinly sliced
1 large onion, peeled, halved and very finely sliced
Salt, freshly ground black pepper and nutmeg
(DF) margarine

1 plump clove of garlic, peeled and crushed
A few thyme leaves
300ml/10fl oz/1 1/4 cups of (GF) vegetable stock
   (bouillon)
Cayenne pepper

Preheat the oven to 180°C/350°F/Gas mark 4

Layer the celeriac with the onion in an ovenproof dish, sprinkling each layer with salt, pepper and nutmeg, and dotting with margarine, garlic and thyme leaves. Continue until all of the celeriac and onion have been used up.

Pour the stock (bouillon) over and sprinkle cayenne pepper over the top.

Bake in the oven until crispy on top and soft all the way through, about 2 hours.

Check occasionally – if it looks as though it is starting to dry out add a little more stock.

Serve the Celeriac Dauphinoise piping hot.

Roast Squash, Chestnuts and Sweet Potatoes

This is a robust accompaniment to roast turkey, pheasant or grouse, especially at Christmas time. It is also unusual and delicious with roast pork or wild boar.

Serves 6–8

1 butternut squash, peeled, halved and seeded

1kg/2.2lb/7 cups of sweet potatoes, peeled (1.5kg/3.3lb for 8 people or more)

200ml/7fl oz/¾ cup of olive oil

Salt and freshly ground black pepper

A little sprinkling of grated cloves and nutmeg

12 whole cloves

225g/8oz/1½ cups of whole peeled chestnuts

Preheat the oven to 180°C/350°F/Gas mark 4

Cut the squash and the potatoes into equal size pieces so that they will take a uniform time to cook. Bring a large pan of water to the boil and blanch the vegetables for 3 minutes in the boiling water. Refresh under cold water and leave to dry for 10 minutes.

Brush the squash and potato pieces with oil and spread them evenly over an oiled baking sheet. Season with salt, pepper, grated cloves and nutmeg and then sprinkle with the whole cloves. Roast in the oven for about 1½ hours. Add the chestnuts 15 minutes before the end so that they heat through.

Serve straight from the oven and remind everyone not to eat the cloves!

Sweet Potato and Orange Purée

In order to be able to enjoy my own dinner parties, I usually prepare the vegetables in the morning and cook them in the microwave as the meat is being carved. No steam, splashes or smells is the essence of a good dinner party in my tiny kitchen.

Serves 6–8

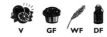

1.5kg/3.3lb/10½ cups of sweet potatoes, peeled and chopped

The grated rind and juice of 2 large oranges

Salt and freshly ground black pepper to taste

1 heaped tablespoon of (DF) margarine

Freshly grated nutmeg to taste

Remove any blemishes from the potatoes and then cook in boiling salted water for 20 minutes or until very soft. Turn off the heat and drain them. Return to the saucepan and mash the potatoes with all of the remaining ingredients until light and fluffy and without lumps. Transfer to a warm serving dish and keep warm until needed.

CHAPTER 3

Pizza, Pasta and Risotto

Chorizo and Artichoke Pizza

Intoxicating, hot and spicy – Spanish or Portuguese sausage is so versatile, eaten cold with a glass of chilled port, or sizzling on a pizza.

Serves 4

BASE

14g/¹/₂oz/1 package of easy-bake yeast or fast-action
   dried yeast
2 teaspoons of caster (superfine) sugar
300ml/10fl oz/1¹/₄ cups of warm water
400g/14oz/2³/₄ cups of (GF) or (WF) flour
¹/₄ teaspoon of salt
Extra (WF) flour for dusting and kneading

TOPPING

2 cloves of garlic, peeled and crushed
1 small red chilli, seeded and chopped
2 tablespoons of olive oil
425g/15oz/2 cups of canned chopped tomatoes,
   excess liquid drained off

2 tablespoons of tomato purée (paste)
A handful of fresh basil leaves, shredded
Salt and freshly ground black pepper
140g/5oz/1¹/₃ cups of chorizo sausages, skinned and
   sliced
400g/14oz of canned artichoke hearts, drained and
   halved
A sprinkling of cayenne pepper
Optional: 250g/9oz carton of virtually fat-free
   cottage cheese or grated reduced-fat mozzarella
   for low-fat toppings, which are not dairy-free or
   a sprinkling of low-fat goat's or sheep's cheese if
   you can tolerate either of them

2 large, non-stick baking trays

Preheat the oven to 200°C/400°F/Gas mark 6

Dissolve the easy-bake yeast, sugar and hot water together in a large jug and whisk thoroughly. Leave in a warm place until the surface is covered with about 2cm/³/₄ inch of froth, about 10–15 minutes, then whisk again. Alternatively, follow the instructions on the packet of fast-action dried yeast but do add the sugar.

Sift the flour and salt together in a large bowl. Beat in the liquid with a wooden spoon and bring the dough together into a ball. To do this, you may need to add a little more warm water until the dough is malleable (different flours absorb varying amounts of water).

Turn the dough onto a floured board and knead with floured hands for 6–10 minutes until the dough is smooth. Spray or lightly grease a large bowl with a little olive oil, place the pizza dough in it and cover with a plate or another bowl. Leave the bowl in a draft-free, very warm area until the dough has doubled in size. This can take 1–2 hours depending on the temperature of your room. Meanwhile, make the topping. Place the garlic, chopped chilli and oil in a saucepan and cook for a second or two. Stir in the tomatoes and tomato purée (paste) and simmer for 5 minutes.

Stir in the basil, salt and pepper and remove from the heat. Cover the saucepan with a lid. Place the pizza dough on a floured board and flatten with a rolling pin. Divide it into 4 portions.

Roll out each portion on a floured board into a thin 20cm/8 inch circle. Place the pizzas on the baking trays. Push each pizza gently outwards with your fingers and pinch up the edges to make a rim and a neat circle.

Cover each pizza with the tomato topping and sprinkle with the chorizo and the artichoke halves. Top the pizzas with the cheese, if using, and then sprinkle the cayenne over them. Bake the pizzas for about 10 minutes or until they are golden brown and crispy and the cheese is bubbling. Carefully slide the pizzas onto hot plates and serve immediately.

Char-grilled Chicken Pasta With Pesto

Hopelessly addicted to fresh coriander (cilantro), I have deviously incorporated it into most of my favourite recipes. In this dish I have used it in place of the more traditional basil in the pesto sauce.

Serves 6

300ml/10fl oz/1¼ cups of olive oil

3 fresh rosemary sprigs, halved

4 chicken breasts, skin on

500g/17oz/6 cups of corn or rice (GF) pasta tubes

1 large bunch (55g/2oz/4 cups) of fresh coriander (cilantro)

30g/1oz/½ cup of fresh parsley

1 clove of garlic, peeled and crushed

100g/3½oz/¾ cup of pine nuts , ground in a food processor

Salt and freshly ground black pepper

Brush a char-grill pan with a little of the oil. Place the rosemary and chicken breasts in the pan and cook until the chicken is crispy and cooked through (about 10 minutes). Discard the skin, then slice the chicken breasts diagonally into bite size pieces. Discard the rosemary.

While the chicken is cooking, boil the pasta in a pan of salted water until just tender. Drain and refresh under hot water. Toss in a bowl with one tablespoon of the olive oil. Mix in the chicken pieces.

In a food processor, blend the remaining oil with the coriander (cilantro), parsley, garlic and pine nuts until smooth. Stir the coriander (cilantro) pesto sauce into the pasta, adjust the seasoning if necessary, and serve immediately.

Gnocchi with Walnut and Lemon Sauce

This was a fun and economical dish that we adored making in Lucca (Italy) when we were staying in the mountains during spring.

Serves 4 (or 6 as a starter)

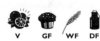

SAUCE

3 large cloves of garlic, peeled and crushed
(GF) chilli oil and extra virgin olive oil to taste
100g/3¹/₂oz/³/₄ cup of finely chopped walnuts
Grated rind and juice of 3 large lemons
2 teaspoons of caster (superfine) sugar
Salt and freshly ground black pepper
15g/¹/₂oz/¹/₄ cup of chopped fresh parsley

GNOCCHI

1kg/2.2lb/7 cups of floury potatoes
1 large free-range egg
200g/7oz/scant ¹/₂ cups of potato flour
85g/3oz/¹/₃ cup of (DF) margarine
15g/¹/₂oz/¹/₂ cup of chopped oregano leaves
Freshly ground black pepper

Extra flour for dusting
1 teaspoon of salt
15g/¹/₂oz/¹/₂ cup of shredded fresh basil leaves

First make the sauce. Cook the garlic in olive oil mixed with the chilli oil (8 tablespoons for 4 people, or 12 tablespoons for 6 people) for a few seconds. Stir in the walnuts and lemon rind and cook for a few more seconds. Add the lemon juice and sugar, salt, pepper and parsley. Keep the sauce warm.

Now make the gnocchi. Peel the potatoes and boil until soft enough to mash. Drain and mash with all the gnocchi ingredients. Allow to cool.

Dust your hands with flour and shape the mixture into walnut size pieces. When the pieces are the correct shape and size, press the back of a fork a little way into the gnocchi to slightly indent and decorate.

Bring a very large pan of water to the boil with a teaspoon of salt and then drop the gnocchi into the water in batches and cook for just 30 seconds. Drain and keep warm in a serving dish.

Pour the sauce over the gnocchi. Serve piping hot, sprinkled with the shredded basil leaves.

Crab Cream Fettuccini

Fresh or frozen crab is always available in good supermarkets so you can serve this pasta any time of the year with a tossed green salad, or stir-fried sugar-snaps and dwarf (green) beans.

Serves 4

---

2 orange peppers, cored and seeded
375g/12 ½ oz/4 ½ cups of corn and parsley (GF) fettuccini
1 tablespoon of olive oil
1 clove of garlic, peeled and chopped
1 bunch of spring onions (scallions), trimmed and sliced
1 mild red chilli, seeded and chopped
2 stems of lemon grass, trimmed and finely chopped

455g/16oz/2 ½ cups of fresh or frozen prepared crab meat
Salt and freshly ground black pepper
The juice of 1 lemon
200ml/7fl oz/¾ cup of coconut cream
Extra oil
1 tablespoon finely chopped coriander (cilantro) leaves

First, finely slice the peppers. Then cook the pasta following the packet's instructions in boiling salted water. Meanwhile, heat the oil in a wok and stir-fry the peppers until slightly softened, then add the garlic, onions, chilli and lemon grass and cook for a couple of minutes. Stir in the crab meat and season with salt and pepper. Mix in the lemon juice and then the coconut cream. Bring to the boil and remove from the heat.

Drain and refresh the pasta under hot water and then return to the pan. Toss in extra oil, salt and pepper.

Serve the pasta immediately on hot plates with the crab cream and sprinkle with coriander (cilantro) leaves.

Seafood Linguine

Now, at last, we can enjoy this fabulous Italian dish with fresh pasta, thanks to The Stamp Collection range of pasta. Sadly, it is not gluten-free but is fabulous for wheat-free gourmets!

Serves 4–6

ULF WF DF

---

1 red onion, peeled and finely chopped

¹/₃ bottle of Italian red wine

340ml/12fl oz/1 ¹/₃ cups carrot or vegetable juice

Salt and freshly ground black pepper

1 medium or hot red chilli, seeded and finely chopped

400g/14oz can of chopped tomatoes

4 bay leaves

1 large sprig of fresh oregano

2 large cloves of garlic, peeled and crushed

1 teaspoon of soft (light) brown sugar

2 × 250g/9oz packets of *The Stamp Collection* (WF) spaghetti

Approximately 900g/2lbs or 6 good handfuls of frozen seafood cocktail, defrosted

A couple of handfuls of fresh basil or fresh parsley leaves to decorate

---

Put the onion, wine, carrot juice, salt, pepper, chilli, tomatoes, bay leaves, oregano, garlic and sugar into a non-stick saucepan and cook over medium heat until the sauce has reduced by about a quarter.

Allow the sauce to cool, remove the bay leaves, then liquidize the sauce to a purée. Return the sauce to the pan and adjust the seasoning to taste.

Bring a large pan of salted water to the boil and cook the spaghetti over high heat until *al dente*. Drain and refresh under hot water, then transfer to a large, warm serving bowl.

Meanwhile, add the seafood to the sauce and simmer for a few minutes until heated through. Shred the basil leaves or chop up the parsley.

Once again, adjust the seasoning of the seafood sauce and then pour over the waiting pasta, sprinkle with the basil or parsley and serve immediately.

Red Pepper Spaghetti

This is a great substitute for tomatoes, which I cannot eat because they are too acidic. Add minced meat or poultry for a great Bolognese sauce.

Serves 6

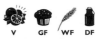

2 onions, peeled and finely chopped

2 tablespoons of olive oil

2 plump cloves of garlic, peeled and crushed

1 plump chilli, seeds removed

Plenty of fresh thyme leaves

4 large red peppers, cored and seeded

1 litre/35fl oz/4 cups of carrot juice

Salt and freshly ground black pepper

600g/21oz/7 cups of (GF) spaghetti (corn, millet or rice only)

Extra olive oil

15g/¹⁄₂oz/¹⁄₂ cup of shredded fresh basil leaves

Cook the onions gently in the oil for 5 minutes and then add the garlic. Chop up the chilli and stir it in with the thyme.

Now chop up the red peppers, add to the onions and cook for 10 minutes until browned in patches only.

Pour in the carrot juice, bring to the boil, then turn down the heat a little and simmer for 30 minutes. Season to taste with salt and pepper. Cool and liquidize.

Cook the spaghetti, following the instructions on the packet. Drain and toss in a little extra olive oil.

Serve immediately on a huge warm dish with the sauce poured over and shredded basil leaves sprinkled on top.

Low-fat Creamy Pasta

I made this pasta dish recently for some American friends of mine who do not eat any fat and are vegetarians. They didn't realise that the fresh pasta I used was gluten free, so that I could indulge too!

Serves 3

V   ULF   WF

1 red onion, peeled and roughly chopped
240ml/8fl oz/1 cup of water
100ml/3½fl oz/½ cup of red wine
1 plump clove of garlic, peeled and crushed
3 stalks of fresh thyme
2 bay leaves
240ml/8fl oz/1 cup of carrot or vegetable juice
1 chilli, seeded and chopped
4 tablespoons of 100% natural pumpkin purée
1 tablespoon of (GF) cornflour (cornstarch) dissolved in 1 tablespoon of water

Salt and freshly ground black pepper
Freshly grated nutmeg
250g/9oz packet of *The Stamp Collection* (WF) fresh spaghetti or other dried varieties available
4–5 tablespoons of virtually fat-free fromage frais or set Greek yogurt
A little freshly chopped parsley and/or grated reduced fat pecorino cheese if allowed!

Place the chopped onion and the water in a non-stick pan and bring to the boil. Drain the onions and refresh them under cold water. Return the onions to the pan with the same amount of fresh water as before and bring to the boil once again.

This time, cook the onions until all the water evaporates.

Add the wine, garlic, thyme and bay leaves to the pan and, stirring frequently, cook for 3–5 minutes until the wine reduces.

Now stir in the carrot juice and chilli and simmer for another 5 minutes. Stir in the pumpkin purée, followed by the dissolved cornflour (cornstarch) and cook for a few minutes. Reduce the heat to low, season to taste with salt, pepper and nutmeg and let the sauce simmer gently while you cook the pasta.

Cook the spaghetti in boiling water for a couple of minutes. Drain it, refresh it under hot water and then return it to the saucepan. Cover with fresh water, bring to the boil again and cook until *al dente*. This prevents the spaghetti becoming sticky and heavy.

Increase the heat slightly under the sauce, add the fromage frais or yogurt to the pan and let it simmer for a couple of minutes, stirring frequently (do not let it boil or the sauce might separate). Drain the cooked spaghetti and transfer it to a warm serving bowl. Pour the hot sauce over the spaghetti and serve immediately, sprinkled with either the chopped parsley or grated pecorino or both.

Red Wine Risotto

This dish, with its deep, rich Burgundy colours, is ideal for a winter lunch or supper with a full-bodied bottle of Italian red wine.

Serves 6

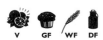

140g/5oz/²/₃ cup of (DF) margarine

2 large red onions, peeled and finely chopped

500g/17oz/2½ cups of risotto rice

600ml/20fl oz/2½ cups of Valpolicella or other fruity full-bodied red wine

Salt and freshly ground black pepper

1 tablespoon of (GF) vegetable stock (bouillon) powder

1 litre/35fl oz/4 cups of boiling water

500g/17oz of ready-cooked, peeled beetroots (beets)

3 tablespoons of chopped fresh parsley

Melt 100g/3½oz/½ cup of the margarine over a medium heat, add the onions and cook gently until nearly soft. Add the rice and stir for a minute. Pour in the red wine and season with salt and pepper. Simmer for 5 minutes.

Mix the stock (bouillon) powder into the water and pour into the rice. Simmer for 10 minutes. Chop up the beetroots (beets) into bite size cubes and stir into the rice. Simmer for 10 more minutes and then fold in the remaining margarine. Adjust the seasoning to taste.

Serve on a large warm dish and sprinkle with chopped parsley.

Spinach and Garlic Risotto

This is simplicity itself and is ideal for lunch, or as a starter. I frequently eat this dish with anchovies dotted all over the top, and a mixed salad.

Serves 6

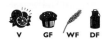

4 tablespoons of olive oil

1 large onion, peeled and finely chopped

2 large cloves of garlic, peeled and crushed

255g/9oz/1¼ cups of arborio rice

500g/17oz/9 cups of fresh or frozen (and defrosted) leaf spinach – do not use chopped spinach

300ml/10fl oz/1¼ cups of dry white vermouth

Salt and freshly ground black pepper

800ml/28fl oz/3⅓ cups of (GF) vegetable stock (bouillon)

The juice of 1 lemon

Grated nutmeg

1 tablespoon of fresh oregano leaves

½ tablespoon of (DF) margarine

Heat the oil and gently cook the onion until soft, but not brown.

Add the garlic. Cook for a moment, then stir in the rice and cook for a few minutes.

Mix in the spinach leaves followed by the vermouth. Season and then pour in the stock (bouillon).

Bring to the boil and simmer for 35 minutes, or until the rice is swollen and soft (top up with water if necessary).

Stir in the lemon juice, nutmeg, oregano and margarine and serve very hot.

This is delicious with grated pecorino (romano) cheese on top.

Sweet Pepper and Courgette Risotto

Courgettes (zucchini) have a high water content and are low in calories. They should always be firm and shiny, not dull and floppy. The bigger the courgette (zucchini) the less flavour it has, so choose small ones, but not the dwarf variety.

Serves 8

V   ULF   GF   WF   DF

1 large red onion, peeled and finely chopped	2 cloves of garlic, peeled and crushed
½ bottle of Italian white wine	Salt and freshly ground black pepper
2 large red peppers, cored and coarsely chopped	1 red chilli, seeded and finely chopped
2 large courgettes (zucchini), trimmed and cut diagonally	1 tablespoon of (GF) vegetable stock (bouillon) powder
170g/6oz/2 cups of your favourite mushrooms, trimmed and thickly sliced	115g/4oz/²/₃ cup of Italian risotto rice
	340ml/12fl oz/1 ⅓ cups of carrot juice
1 large sprig of thyme	A pinch of saffron
1 large sprig of rosemary	A large handful of fresh basil leaves, shredded
4 bay leaves	

Place the onion and wine in a large, non-stick pan and cook over medium heat until the onion softens. Top up with water if the liquid evaporates too quickly.

Add the peppers, courgettes (zucchini), mushrooms, all the herbs, garlic, seasoning and chilli. Cook for about 5 minutes, then add the stock (bouillon) powder, rice, carrot juice, saffron and 600ml/20fl oz/2½ cups of hot water.

Simmer the risotto for about 15 minutes, until most of the liquid is absorbed, then top up with about half again of hot water (different kinds of rice absorb liquids differently, so the amount of water you will need to keep the rice moist will vary). Simmer the rice and vegetables for another 15 minutes or until they are tender. Adjust the seasoning to taste, adding more chilli if you like your risotto highly seasoned.

Stir the risotto from time to time, to prevent it sticking to the bottom of the pan.

Serve the risotto in a warm dish and sprinkle liberally with shredded basil leaves and black pepper.

CHAPTER 4

Fish and Seafood

Grilled Sea Bass with Orange and Vermouth Sauce

Most bass sold in shops has never seen the ocean; like salmon, it is now heavily farmed. Intensively farmed fish have a slightly different texture and taste to wild ones and are fatter but less expensive.

Serves 2

ULF GF WF DF

2 medium-sized (115–170g/4–6oz) sea bass
   steaks, skin on

Salt and freshly ground black pepper

Fresh thyme leaves

1 bulb of fennel, trimmed and tough outer
   layers removed

The juice of 2 oranges and the zest of 1 orange

4 tablespoons of dry white vermouth

4 tablespoons of (GF) vegetable stock (bouillon)

5 spring onions (scallions), trimmed and finely
   chopped

1 tablespoon of (GF) cornflour (cornstarch),
   dissolved in 1 tablespoon of water

Rinse the sea bass in cold water and then, using a sharp knife, make 2–3 small incisions on the side of the fish. Put the sea bass on a plate and sprinkle with a little salt, pepper and fresh thyme leaves (reserving a few for decoration). Leave to rest for 30 minutes in a cool place.

Finely slice the fennel with a very sharp knife and place in a non-stick frying pan (skillet) with the orange juice and zest, the vermouth, stock (bouillon) and spring onions (scallions). Bring to the boil, reduce the heat and simmer until the fennel pieces are nearly soft. Stir in the dissolved cornflour (cornstarch), bring the sauce to the boil again, turn down the heat and stir the sauce until it is clear and thickened. Keep the pan of fennel on low heat while you cook the fish.

Preheat the grill (broiler) to the hottest setting and cook the fish, skin side up, for about 5 minutes. The quicker the fish cooks, the juicier the flesh will be under the seared skin.

Pour the fennel sauce onto 2 warm plates and place the sea bass in the centre. Decorate with a couple of sprigs of fresh thyme and serve immediately with baby new potatoes and fresh, crunchy green vegetables.

Roast Halibut on Beetroot and Cumin Purée

This lively and colourful dish, full of spices and herbs, reminds me of the Polish soup Borsch. If you use fresh beetroots (beets) the flavour will be stronger, but I am normally so busy that I cheat and use ready-cooked and prepared ones instead.

Serves 2

ULF GF WF

1 large potato, peeled and cubed	240ml/8fl oz/1 cup of cold water
2 tablespoons of skimmed milk	2 bay leaves
Salt and freshly ground black pepper	2 freshly prepared halibut steaks (choose size
4 medium-sized, ready-cooked and prepared	according to appetite!)
beetroots (beets)	A large sprig of fresh thyme
1 clove fresh garlic, peeled and crushed	1/2 a lemon, freshly squeezed
1 teaspoon of (GF) vegetable stock (bouillon) powder	1 lemon, cut into quarters
1/2 teaspoon of ground cumin	Fresh thyme sprigs to decorate
1/2 teaspoon of (GF) mixed (pie) spice	

First make the beetroot (beet) and cumin purée. Cook the potato in boiling water until soft, then mash with the skimmed milk and season with salt and pepper. Chop the beetroots (beets) and put them into a saucepan with the garlic, stock (bouillon) powder, cumin, mixed spice and the cold water. Bring to the boil and simmer for 10 minutes.

Leave the mixture to cool slightly, then purée it in a food processor. (The purée must be very thick otherwise the mash will be too runny to take the weight of the fish. If it is too runny, return it to a non-stick pan and simmer until it has reduced and thickened.)

Mix the purée into the mashed potatoes and stir the mixture until it is an even texture and colour throughout. Adjust the seasoning according to taste.

Place the beetroot (beet) and potato mixture in a non-stick pan and heat through over a gentle heat until needed.

Put the two bay leaves on a non-stick baking tray and place the portions of halibut on top. Sprinkle the fish with the thyme leaves, salt, pepper and some of the lemon juice. Grill (broil) the fish for a few minutes under very high heat so that the juices are sealed in. Turn the halibut over and grill (broil) until just cooked through.

Place the hot purée in the centre of each plate and place the fish on top, removing the bay leaf first! Serve with the lemon segments and decorate with sprigs of fresh thyme.

Plaice in Tomato and Basil Hollandaise

Thick fillets of fish are successfully roasted in the oven at a very high temperature. This produces crispy skin and juicy flesh inside.

Serves 4

GF / WF DF

4 whole plaice, filleted into halves
Sunflower oil
Salt and freshly ground black pepper
I tablespoon of dry white vermouth

TOMATO AND BASIL
HOLLANDAISE
170g/6oz/³/4 cup of (DF) margarine
4 large free-range egg yolks
I tablespoon of water
I tablespoon of lemon juice
Salt and freshly ground black pepper
340g/12oz/2 cups of tomatoes, fresh or canned,
  skinned, drained and finely chopped
15g/¹/2oz/¹/2 cup of basil leaves, shredded

Extra basil leaves for decoration

Preheat the oven to 200°C/400°F/Gas mark 6

Brush the plaice with a little oil, season, sprinkle over the vermouth and bake for about 5 minutes on a non-stick roasting tray.
Next, make the hollandaise sauce. Put the margarine into a saucepan and bring to the boil.
Put the egg yolks, water, lemon juice, salt and pepper into a food processor and blend briefly.
As soon as the margarine comes to the boil, turn on the food processor and pour the margarine into the machine, continuing to blend until the sauce is thick. Turn off the processor and add the tomatoes and basil leaves. Adjust the seasoning if necessary. Pour the sauce into a bowl.
Serve the plaice on a warm plate with a pool of sauce and sprinkle with extra basil leaves.

Ocean Pie

This is all seafood and fish and omits the more traditional eggs, therefore is quicker to make and rather more French!

Serves 6–8

GF WF DF

600ml/20fl oz/2 ½ cups of ready-made (GF) fish stock
  (bouillon)
1 small red onion, peeled and finely chopped
½ a lemon
1 teaspoon of fresh thyme leaves
1 bay leaf
950g/2lb/5 ½ cups of cod fillet, skinned and boned
400g/14oz/3 ½ cups of frozen seafood, defrosted
200ml/7fl oz/¾ cup of dry white vermouth
100g/3 ½ oz/7 tablespoons of (DF) margarine

55g/2oz/scant ½ cup of rice flour
240ml/8fl oz/1 cup of soya cream
Salt and freshly ground black pepper
15g/½ oz/½ cup of fresh dill, chopped
1kg/2.2lb/7 cups of potatoes, peeled and trimmed
1 small whole celeriac, peeled and blemishes
  removed
Grated nutmeg
Extra margarine and some cayenne pepper

Preheat the oven to 200°C/400°F/Gas mark 6

Place the stock (bouillon) in a pan and add the onion, lemon, thyme and bay leaf. Bring to the boil and cook for 10 minutes.

Chop the cod into bite size pieces. Reduce the heat, discard the lemon then add the cod and seafood.

Add the vermouth and poach gently for 3 minutes. Leave to cool away from the heat.

Melt half of the margarine in a large saucepan and beat in the flour. Gradually incorporate the vermouth stock.

Drain the fish, reserving the juices, then slowly beat the fish juices into the sauce until it is thick and smooth. Bring to the boil and cook for 1 minute, stirring all the time. Blend in the soya cream and seafood and season with salt, pepper and dill. Leave to one side.

Chop the potato and celeriac into small chunks and then cook in salted boiling water until very soft. Drain and return to the pan with the remaining margarine and salt, pepper and nutmeg to taste and mash until smooth. Spoon the fish and sauce into a deep ovenproof dish and smooth the mash over it. Dot with a little extra margarine and a sprinkling of cayenne pepper and bake for 20 minutes. Serve straight from the oven.

Vodka Lime Seafood Salad

Beware of drinking and driving. The powerful kick this dish has could take you over the limit! The vodka softens the fish, so it melts in your mouth.

Serves 4

GF / WF / DF

600g/21 oz/3¹/₂ cups of very fresh, or frozen, haddock fillets, skinned and boned

1 large mild red chilli, halved and seeded

¹/₂ a small red onion, peeled and finely chopped

170g/6oz/1¹/₂ cups of very fresh prawns (shrimp), shells removed

Salt and freshly ground black pepper

The juice of 1 large lemon

The grated rind and juice of 3 limes

4 tablespoons of vodka

2 tablespoons of chilli olive oil or olive oil

40g/1¹/₂ oz of prepared lamb's lettuce (mâche)

A handful of coriander (cilantro) leaves to garnish

Cut the fish into attractive slender lengths and finely chop the chilli.

Mix the fish and chilli with the onion, prawns (shrimp), salt and pepper, lemon juice, rind and juice of the limes, vodka and chilli oil and leave to marinate for 2–4 hours, or overnight, in a shallow dish under clingfilm (plastic wrap).

Arrange the fish salad and all its juices on a serving plate with the lamb's lettuce (mâche) and sprinkle with a little chopped coriander (cilantro).

Alternatively, serve the salad on individual plates with slices of (GF) sourdough bread to mop up the juices.

Tuna Fish Carpaccio with Mint and Caper Salad

It has recently been claimed that eating fresh tuna twice a week has helped some people with stiff joints to feel more mobile. Tuna is an oily fish – which is no doubt why it might help ease stiff joints – but in this recipe the fat content is kept very low by serving it in wafer thin slices with an oil-free dressing. This dish must be ultra fresh otherwise it is not worth making.

Serves 4

ULF GF WF DF

2–4 wafer thin slices of fresh fillet of tuna per person

85g/3oz/4 handfuls of fresh rocket (arugula) leaves

Salt and freshly ground black pepper

1 mild red chilli, seeded and finely chopped

5 spring onions (scallions), trimmed and finely sliced

4 small fresh plum tomatoes, skinned, seeded and finely chopped

1 small cucumber, peeled, halved lengthways and seeded

1 heaped teaspoon of (GF) Dijon mustard

2 tablespoons of red wine vinegar

1/2 clove of garlic, peeled and crushed

A handful of chopped fresh mint leaves

2 tablespoons of good quality capers (not in malt vinegar)

Grated zest of 1 large lemon

Juice of 1 large orange

A small bunch of fresh parsley, chopped

Ask the fishmonger to slice the tuna into wafer thin slices for you or do it yourself using a very sharp knife.

Arrange the rocket (arugula) leaves on four large plates. Place the tuna slices on the salad leaves and season it all with a little pepper.

In a bowl, mix the chilli with the onions and tomatoes and season to taste with salt and pepper. Chop the cucumber into tiny pieces and add to the bowl of tomatoes. Stir in the mustard, followed by the vinegar and garlic. Now mix in the chopped mint, capers, lemon zest and orange juice and stir gently until it is blended.

If you find the dressing too strong, then add a teaspoon of water at a time until the taste is to your liking.

Spoon the salad and juices over the tuna carpaccio and sprinkle with the chopped parsley.

Serve with baby new potatoes.

Fresh Tuna and Quails' Egg Salad Niçoise

A perfect main course for the summer, easy to prepare and to transport outside with a couple of cool bottles of wine and fresh (GF) bread to mop up the dressing.

Serves 6 (or 12 as a starter)

GF   WF   DF

1kg/2.2lb/7 cups of baby new potatoes, scrubbed

600g/21oz/7 cups of French dwarf (green) beans, topped and tailed

24 baby tomatoes, wiped and halved

1 small red onion, very finely sliced

24 black olives, stoned (pitted)

3 tablespoons of chopped fresh parsley

Salt and freshly ground black pepper

24 quails' eggs, hard boiled for 3 minutes in boiling water, then transferred to cold water

12 anchovy fillets, drained and halved

3 tablespoons of virgin olive oil

2 tablespoons of lemon juice

1 large clove of garlic, peeled and crushed

6 large fresh tuna steaks or 12 small

Extra olive oil

Cook the potatoes in salted boiling water until just soft. Drain and put in a large dish.

Cook the beans, ensuring that they remain crunchy. Drain and refresh under cold water and mix with the potatoes.

Now add the tomatoes, onion, olives, half the parsley, salt and pepper. Peel and halve the eggs and mix into the salad. Add the anchovies.

Mix the oil, lemon juice and garlic together and sprinkle all over the salad.

Finally, brush the tuna fish with a little oil and grill (broil) or char-grill until just cooked through. Place each steak on a bed of salad, sprinkle with the remaining parsley and serve or chill until needed.

For a more economical alternative, cook 540g/18oz of fresh tuna then flake the flesh into the salad.

Grilled Scallops with Sage and Capers

In Italy, the caper is a delight; large, plump, mellow and juicy – quite unlike the minute offerings we get here in England. The very best capers are grown in Salina, an island off the coast of Sicily. Rather than being drowned in sharp vinegar, they are dried in high quality sea salt, which removes the bitterness and draws out the complex flavours.

Serves 1–2

ULF   GF   WF   DF

255g/9oz/1⅓ cups of scallops with their corals
6–8 fresh sage leaves, chopped
1 clove of garlic, peeled and crushed
Salt and freshly ground black pepper
4 tablespoons of water

2 heaped tablespoons of high quality capers
   (not in malt vinegar), drained
4 tablespoons of Marsala
1 heaped tablespoon of chopped fresh parsley

Place the scallops, sage, garlic, seasoning, water and capers in a non-stick frying pan (skillet) and cook for a 2–3 minutes. Add the Marsala and cook the scallops for another couple of minutes. Shake the pan from time to time so that the scallops are evenly cooked through.

Remove the scallops from the pan and place on 2 warm plates.

Quickly boil up the juices in the pan for 1–2 minutes. Pour the sauce over the scallops and decorate with a sprinkling of chopped fresh parsley.

Serve at once with warm fresh bread and a wonderful mixed green salad with fresh herbs.

Stuffed Squid in Red Wine Sauce

Stuffing squid and serving it in a rich sauce is a good way of making this light seafood into a substantial main course. Don't forget that squid needs only brief cooking, otherwise it will become tough and chewy.

Serves 2

ULF GF WF DF

2 heaped tablespoons of risotto rice

16 whole cleaned squid with their tentacles

1 small red onion, peeled and very finely chopped

2 teaspoons of mixed herbs

600ml/20fl oz/2½ cups of (GF) vegetable or fish stock (bouillon)

Salt and freshly ground black pepper

Freshly grated nutmeg

1 large clove of garlic, peeled and crushed

⅓ bottle of good Italian red wine

225g/8oz or 3 large flat mushrooms

200ml/7fl oz/¾ cup of (GF) vegetable or fish stock (bouillon)

100ml/3½ fl oz/scant ½ cup of dry sherry

1 heaped tablespoon of tomato purée (paste)

1 heaped tablespoon of finely chopped sun-dried tomatoes

1 mild chilli, seeded and finely chopped

1 tablespoon of (GF) cornflour (cornstarch), dissolved in 1 tablespoon of water

A handful of fresh parsley, finely chopped

First cook the rice in salted, boiling water until just soft. Drain, rinse under hot water and set aside. Wash the squid in cold water, drain, remove the tentacles and keep in a cool place until needed. Place half the chopped onion, 1 teaspoon of the mixed herbs, the stock (bouillon), salt and pepper, nutmeg, garlic and red wine in a large non-stick pan and bring to the boil. Reduce the heat and simmer it until the liquid is reduced by one third.

Chop the mushrooms into fairly large pieces (if using small, wild mushrooms keep them whole). Add the mushrooms to the red wine sauce and simmer for about 3 minutes.

Now make the stuffing. Cook the other onion half in the stock (bouillon) and sherry until soft. Add the cooked rice and the remaining teaspoon of mixed herbs and simmer for a few minutes. Meanwhile, choose 6 of the smallest squid bodies, finely chop them and add them to the rice along with the tomato purée (paste), sun-dried tomato pieces and chilli. Cook for another 5 minutes or until the squid is just white and the rice is moist but not wet or dry. Adjust the seasoning to taste with salt, pepper and grated nutmeg and remove the rice from the heat.

When the rice mixture is cool enough to handle, carefully pack it into each of the squid using your fingertips. Fill the body up, squeeze the mixture down to the end and level it off.

Bring the wine sauce back to simmering point over medium heat, stir in the dissolved cornflour (cornstarch) and bring to the boil. Once the sauce has thickened, turn down the heat and place all the stuffed squid and the tentacles in the sauce. Cook the squid over medium heat for a few minutes before turning them over. Simmer only until the squid are cooked through, then serve them immediately with a sprinkling of fresh parsley. Serve with a delicious continental salad of herbs, mixed lettuce leaves and fresh vine tomatoes.

Grilled Salmon on Puy Lentils

Well-produced farmed salmon is perfectly good but wild salmon is wonderful and as full of character as the fishermen who catch it.

Serves 4

2 tablespoons of chilli olive oil

1 tablespoon of fresh thyme leaves

1 large red onion, peeled and finely chopped

247g/8oz/1⅓ cups of canned puy lentils, drained (or 247g/8oz/1⅓ cups of dried puy lentils, cooked for 45 minutes instead of 8 minutes)

2 large cloves of garlic, peeled and crushed

Salt and freshly ground pepper

1 tablespoon of balsamic vinegar

300ml/10fl oz/1¼ cups of water

3 tablespoons of chopped parsley

3 tablespoons of dry sherry

A little olive oil

4 × 200g/7oz salmon steaks

1 tablespoon of (DF) margarine

Place the chilli olive oil and thyme leaves in a frying pan (skillet), add the onion and cook the onion gently until it is soft.

Add the lentils, garlic, salt and pepper and lastly the vinegar. Simmer for 8 minutes, adding the water as soon as the mixture starts to stick. Stir in half the parsley and the sherry, adding more water if necessary.

In another pan, fry the salmon steaks in a little olive oil until crispy on the outside and slightly underdone inside. Stir the margarine into the lentils.

Spoon a pool of lentils in juices onto each plate and serve with the salmon nesting on top.

Sprinkle with the remaining parsley and enjoy it with a watercress salad or mashed potatoes.

Steamed Cod on Mint Purée

Cod is such an underrated fish and so I have decided to glamorize it to dinner party level!

Serves 4

1kg/2.2lb/8³/4 cups of baby broad (fava) beans, defrosted

650g/23oz/4¹/2 cups of potatoes, peeled and chopped

2 large free-range egg yolks

55g/2oz/¹/4 cup of (DF) margarine

750g/26oz fillet of fresh cod, skinned and boned

The juice of 1¹/2 lemons

Salt and freshly ground black pepper

Freshly grated nutmeg

1 clove of garlic, peeled and crushed

2 tablespoons of soya cream

15g/¹/2 oz/¹/2 cup of fresh mint leaves, finely chopped

A little olive oil and a few extra mint leaves

40g/1¹/2 oz/¹/2 cup of fresh rocket (arugula) leaves

First, cook the broad (fava) beans in salted, boiling water for 4 minutes. Drain and refresh under cold water. Cook the potatoes in salted boiling water until soft.

Meanwhile, peel all the skins off the broad (fava) beans and discard. Drain the potatoes and mash with the egg yolks and margarine until smooth.

Sprinkle the cod with one third of the lemon juice, season with salt and pepper and steam or grill it until it is just cooked through.

Purée the broad (fava) beans in a food processor with one third of the lemon juice, salt, pepper, nutmeg, garlic and soya cream. Beat this mixture into the mashed potatoes, adding the chopped mint. Adjust the seasoning. Divide the purée between 4 warm plates. Put the cooked fish on top and sprinkle with the remaining lemon juice and the extra mint leaves to decorate.

Serve immediately, surrounded with rocket (arugula) leaves and drizzled with a little olive oil and black pepper.

Roast Swordfish with Basil

Swordfish has become very trendy and is now sold in most large supermarkets.

Serves 4

4 swordfish steaks, about 750g/26oz total weight

1 tablespoon of olive oil

Salt and freshly ground black pepper

400g/14oz/2 cups of butter (lima) beans, drained

2 tablespoons of chilli olive oil

1 large chilli, seeded and finely chopped

8 spring onions (scallions), trimmed and finely sliced

Lots of fresh basil, shredded

1 very large tomato, skinned, seeded and chopped

Preheat the oven to 200°C/400°F/Gas mark 6

Brush the swordfish with the oil, sprinkle with salt and pepper and leave on a non-stick baking sheet for a moment. Cook the butter (lima) beans gently in the chilli oil with the chilli and spring onions (scallions) for 5 minutes.

Now put the fish in the oven. Add a little of the chopped basil to the beans, then add the chopped tomato and simmer for 5 minutes, by which time the fish will be cooked. Season the beans to taste.

Serve the fish steaks on hot plates with a large spoonful of beans sprinkled with the remaining fresh basil to decorate.

Smoked Haddock and Mushroom Roulade

This is a fun way of cooking haddock, which can be made into a party piece by using exotic wild mushrooms instead of shiitake.

Serves 4–6 (Optional)

GF / WF DF

340g/12oz of smoked haddock fillet, skinned and boned

300ml/10fl oz/1¼ cups of soya milk

2 large bay leaves

115g/4oz/½ cup of (DF) margarine

30g/1oz/scant ¼ cup of rice flour

2 teaspoons of mild (GF/DF) curry paste or powder

4 large free-range eggs, separated

Salt and freshly ground black pepper

3 tablespoons of grated pecorino (romano) or Etorki cheese (if sheep's cheese is tolerated), or

3 tablespoons chopped nuts, lightly browned in oven

Cayenne pepper

225g/8oz/3 cups of shiitake mushrooms, sliced

Grated nutmeg

6 tablespoons of soya cream

25 x 36cm/10 x 14 inch roulade tin, carefully lined with greased baking parchment (wax paper)

Preheat the oven to 200°C/400°F/Gas mark 6

Poach the haddock in the milk with the bay leaves, until just cooked. Flake the fish as soon as it is cool enough. Discard the bay leaves and reserve the milk.

Make a roux with half the margarine, melting it in a non-stick saucepan and gradually beating in the flour and curry paste. Beat in the reserved milk and cook until smooth and thick. Cool and beat in the fish and egg yolks. Season to taste with salt and pepper.

In another bowl, whisk the egg whites until stiff. Fold 1 spoonful into the fish, then gently fold the rest in with a metal spoon. Tip this into the tin, spread evenly and bake for 15–20 minutes until firm.

Cool for a few minutes and then tip onto a large piece of baking parchment (wax paper) that has been scattered with sheep's cheese, nuts or just a little cayenne pepper. Peel away the paper from the roulade and discard. Slice off both ends of the roulade if they are a little dry. Cover the roulade with a clean tea towel.

Now melt the remaining margarine and cook the mushrooms for a few minutes. Season with salt, pepper and nutmeg. Stir in the cream and remove from the heat. Remove the cloth and lift the roulade onto a warm serving dish. Spread the mushroom filling all over it and, using the paper underneath to help you, roll up the roulade. Pull off the paper and serve the roulade immediately with a green salad.

Quick Salmon Soufflé

Soufflés are cheap and easy – ideal for supper with a salad or as an enterprising starter.

Serves 3

GF WF DF

200g/7oz of fresh salmon fillets
1 tablespoon of very dry white vermouth
Salt and freshly ground black pepper
1 heaped tablespoon of (DF) margarine
2 heaped tablespoons of rice flour
3 tablespoons of soya cream
3 large free-range egg yolks, beaten

Grated nutmeg
5 egg whites
Cayenne pepper

A large soufflé dish, greased with (DF) margarine
  and coated with 2 tablespoons of (GF)
  breadcrumbs

Preheat the oven to 200°C/400°F/Gas mark 6

Poach the salmon in a little water with the vermouth, salt and freshly ground black pepper until just cooked through. Cool, then remove the skin and bones and flake the fish, reserving the poaching liquid.

Melt the margarine in a non-stick saucepan and beat in the flour. Add the poaching liquid and then the salmon.

Beat until smooth and thick. Bring to the boil and cook for 1 minute. Remove from the heat. Add the soya cream and egg yolks and mix well. Season with pepper and nutmeg and blend briefly in the food processor until pale pink and smooth. Transfer to a bowl.

In a clean bowl, whisk the eggs with a pinch of salt until firm. Stir one spoonful into the salmon and then quickly and gently fold the rest in with a metal spoon. Spoon into the prepared soufflé dish and sprinkle with cayenne pepper.

Bake for 30–35 minutes until golden, firm and well risen. Serve immediately.

Tuna Fishcakes and Dill Sauce

Corn meal is a brilliant substitute for flour, which is not tolerated by coeliacs, and should satisfy even the most discerning palate.

Serves 6

15g/¹/₂oz/¹/₂ cup of fresh dill, chopped

1 tablespoon of mild (GF) mustard

4 tablespoons of (GF/DF) mayonnaise

3 tablespoons of soya cream

1 tablespoon of olive oil

400g/14oz/2¹/₂ cups of tuna fish in brine, drained

900g/32oz/6 cups of potatoes, peeled, boiled and mashed

Freshly grated nutmeg

Salt and freshly ground black pepper

A dash of (GF) Tabasco sauce/hot chilli oil

1 tablespoon of chopped fresh parsley

1 tablespoon of (DF) margarine

(GF) cornflour (cornstarch) for dusting

2 eggs, beaten

200g/7oz/1¹/₂ cups of fine corn meal

Oil for frying

First, make the sauce by mixing the dill, mustard, mayonnaise, cream and oil. Season to taste, then cover and chill until needed.

Mash the tuna fish with the potatoes and season with nutmeg, salt and pepper, Tabasco sauce and parsley, then beat in the margarine.

Dust your clean hands with cornflour (cornstarch) and roll the mixture into 12 patties. Dip each fishcake into the beaten egg and roll in corn meal. Chill in the deep freeze for half an hour.

Now fry in a little hot oil until crispy and golden, about 5 minutes on each side. Drain briefly on kitchen (paper) towels and serve immediately with the dill sauce.

Thai Coconut Sauté

More and more delicious Asian and Indian spice mixtures and ingredients are appearing in supermarkets so that we can experiment with the flavours we so eagerly devour on holidays abroad.

Serves 2

GF   WF   DF

100g/3¹/₂oz/¹/₂ cup of rice
16 x 6–7cm/2¹/₂ inch prawns (shrimp) in shells, peeled but tails left intact or 200g/7oz/1³/₄ cups of peeled, defrosted prawns (shrimp)
1 large red pepper, cored and finely sliced
1 bunch of spring onions (scallions), trimmed and sliced
1 small mild red chilli, seeded and chopped

1 large clove of garlic, peeled and crushed
1 tablespoon each of sunflower oil and chilli olive oil
2–3 teaspoons of red Thai spice
300ml/10fl oz/1³/₄ cups of coconut milk
Salt and freshly ground black pepper
The juice of 2 limes
1 tablespoon of fresh coriander (cilantro) leaves

Cook the rice in salted, boiling water until tender.

Meanwhile, slit the inside length of the prawns (shrimp) to prevent them curling up too much.

Drain and refresh the rice under hot water and keep warm.

Stir-fry the red pepper, spring onions (scallions), chilli and garlic in the oils in a heated wok over a high heat until softened but not browned. Stir in the red Thai spice and cook for 1 minute. Mix in the coconut milk and season with salt and pepper. Stir in the prawns (shrimp) and the lime juice and cook for a couple of minutes or until the prawns (shrimp) are hot.

Spoon the rice into the centre of two hot plates. Spoon over the prawns (shrimp) and sauce.

Sprinkle with coriander (cilantro) and serve.

CHAPTER 5

Meat Dishes

Steak and Kidney Pudding

Traditional English pub food at its best. The pudding is packed with spices and herbs, so the aroma when it is cut open is wonderful.

Serves 5

FILLING

565g/20oz/2¹/₂ cups of chuck steak, trimmed and
   chopped
285g/10oz/1¹/₄ cups of kidneys of your choice,
   trimmed and chopped
4 tablespoons of well seasoned (GF) flour
2 tablespoons of olive oil
1 onion, peeled and finely sliced
200ml/7fl oz/³/₄ cup of dry sherry
1 tablespoon of (GF) Dijon mustard
1 tablespoon of (GF) Worcestershire sauce
A few drops of (GF) Tabasco sauce
1 teaspoon of (GF) mixed (pie) spice or allspice
3 cloves, and a pinch of grated nutmeg

SUET PASTRY

100g/3¹/₂oz/²/₃ cup of rice flour
100g/3¹/₂oz/²/₃ cup of buckwheat flour
70g/2¹/₂oz/²/₃ cup of potato flour
3 teaspoons of (GF) baking powder
140g/5oz/1 cup of (GF) shredded suet
Salt and freshly ground black pepper
240ml/8fl oz/1 cup of water

1.7 litre/3 pint pudding bowl, oiled
Baking parchment (wax paper)
String

Make the filling first. Toss the steak and kidneys in the flour. Heat the oil in a large pan and cook the onion for 5 minutes until soft, but not brown. Add the meat and seal on all sides. Pour in the sherry, stir in the mustard and Worcestershire sauce, Tabasco sauce, spice, cloves and nutmeg and simmer gently while you make the pastry.

Sift and mix the flours with the baking powder. Fold in the suet, salt and pepper. Now gradually mix in the cold water using a couple of blunt-edged knives. The dough will slowly come together. Use your hands to form the dough into a ball and knead briefly.

Roll out three quarters of the pastry on a floured board into a 35cm/14-inch circle and then line the oiled pudding bowl with it. Quickly pour in the meat filling and then roll out the remaining pastry to cover the top. Seal by pinching the edges with cold water on your finger tips. Pierce the top with a sharp knife.

Cover the top of the pudding with baking parchment (wax paper), making a central pleat by folding it over with plenty of space for the pastry to expand. Tie up with string. Place the bowl on a folded piece of foil in a large saucepan and fill with boiling water to half way up the bowl. Cover the saucepan with a lid or tightly wrapped foil and boil for 2 hours (checking the water level regularly) until the pastry is cooked and the meat is tender.

Lift the pudding bowl out of the saucepan and leave for 5 minutes. Remove the lid and serve the pudding in the bowl, wrapped in a clean white linen napkin.

Beef en Croûte with Tomato and Basil Hollandaise

This recipe can also be made with salmon, lamb, pork or veal. After Christmas, it's a good way of using up leftover turkey breast.

Serves 4

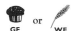

PASTRY

255g/9oz/1¾ cups of (WF) flour or ⅓ each of (GF)
   rice flour, maize flour and potato flour
A good pinch of salt
70g/2½ oz/⅓ cup of (DF) margarine
70g/2½ oz/⅓ cup of lard
1 large free-range egg yolk
4 tablespoons of cold water

BEEF FILLING

400g/14oz/3½ cups of button mushrooms, wiped
   and trimmed of stalks
2 tablespoons of olive oil
1 clove of garlic, peeled and chopped
2 teaspoons of fresh thyme leaves

Salt and freshly ground black pepper
725g/25oz of fillet steak, trimmed
Oil for brushing
½ a beaten egg

TOMATO AND BASIL HOLLANDAISE

340g/12oz/2 cups of tomatoes, fresh or canned,
   skinned, drained and finely chopped
170g/6oz/¾ cup of (DF) margarine
4 large free-range egg yolks
1 tablespoon of water
1 tablespoon of lemon juice
Salt and freshly ground black pepper
15g/½oz/½ cup of basil leaves, shredded

Preheat the oven to 200°C/400°F/Gas mark 6

First, make the pastry. Put the flour into a large bowl and mix in the salt. Add the margarine and lard in pieces and mix with two blunt-edged knives, using one in each hand. Then rub the mixture with your clean finger tips, lifting and crumbling to aerate it. Make a well in the centre, add the egg and water and blend together. Work lightly and wrap in clingfilm (plastic wrap). Chill for 30 minutes.

Fill a bowl with boiling water and immerse the tomatoes for the sauce. Pierce the skin once or twice and leave for 3 minutes, then drain. Now peel off the skin, remove the seeds and chop up the flesh.

Finely slice the mushrooms and cook gently in the 2 tablespoons of oil, garlic and half the thyme. Season to taste and keep to one side.

Brush the beef with oil, season with salt, pepper and the remaining thyme. Divide the dough in half. Sprinkle flour on a board, roll the pastry into a rectangle, and trim with a sharp knife to about 2cm/³/₄ inch larger than the beef. Put half the mushrooms in the centre of the pastry and cover with the beef.

Spoon the remaining mushrooms over the top of the meat. Roll out the other half of the pastry and place over the beef, with a similar overhang of about 2cm/³/₄ inch. Bring both pieces of pastry together and seal by pinching with your fingertips. Decorate with a few cut-out pastry leaves or flowers according to your artistic talents! Brush with beaten egg.

Very gently criss-cross the pastry with a blunt-edged knife and make a little incision in the centre to let the air escape. Bake in the oven for 35 minutes until golden.

While this is baking, make the Hollandaise sauce. Put the margarine into a saucepan and bring to the boil. Meanwhile, put the egg yolks, water, lemon juice, salt and pepper into a food processor and blend briefly.

As soon as the margarine comes to the boil, turn on the food processor and pour the margarine into the machine. Continue to blend until the sauce is thick. Turn off the processor and add the tomatoes and basil leaves. Transfer the sauce to a warm serving bowl.

Carve the fillet into thick slices and serve with a pool of sauce. Crunchy broccoli and French beans balance the dish very nicely.

Beef Casserole with Dumplings

Use a rich, fruity red wine like Barolo from Italy and the casserole will be meltingly tender and full of flavour.

Serves 6

BEEF CASSEROLE

1kg/2.2lb of stewing steak

2 tablespoons of seasoned (GF) cornflour (cornstarch)

2 tablespoons of olive oil

30g/1oz/2 tablespoons of (DF) margarine

1 large onion, peeled and sliced

125g/4½oz/⅔ cup of unsmoked streaky bacon, cut into strips

1 large carrot, finely chopped

2 stalks of celery, finely chopped

3 tablespoons of chopped fresh parsley

12 sage leaves, chopped

2 bay leaves

1 sprig of rosemary

3 cloves of garlic, peeled and crushed

Freshly grated nutmeg

Salt and freshly ground black pepper

1 bottle of Barolo, or a full-bodied red wine

225g/8oz/2½ cups of mushrooms of any kind, in quarters or halves, according to size

DUMPLINGS

55g/2oz/scant ½ cup of buckwheat flour

55g/2oz/scant ½ cup of rice flour

70g/2½oz/½ cup of potato flour

2 heaped teaspoons of (GF) baking powder

Salt and freshly ground black pepper

3 tablespoons of chopped parsley

70g/2½oz/½ cup of (GF) shredded suet

Preheat the oven to 150°C/300°F/Gas mark 2

Cut the steak into bite size pieces and coat in the seasoned flour. Place the oil and margarine in a casserole dish, add the steak and fry until lightly browned.

Add the onion and bacon and fry for a further couple of minutes. Stir in the carrot, celery, all the herbs, garlic and seasoning.

Mix in the red wine and cover. Transfer to the oven and simmer for 2 hours.

While the casserole is cooking, make the dumplings. First, mix the flours and baking powder, salt, pepper and parsley together in a bowl. Blend in the suet, but do not rub it in. Add just enough cold water to make a dough. Knead very lightly and shape into 12 dumplings.

Half an hour before the end of cooking time, add the mushrooms to the casserole, then place the dumplings all over the surface. Bake, uncovered, for the last half hour until the dumplings are golden and crusty.

Serve piping hot with Celeriac Dauphinoise (*see page 33*).

Lamb Dauphinoise

A layer of browned, sliced celeriac tops this mince dish and transforms it into easy, flexible party food. You can use any kind of mince: turkey, venison or veal are the less fattening options.

Serves 6

GF / WF / DF

SAUCE

400g/14oz/1¾ cups of natural soya yogurt (or Greek-style set sheep's yogurt, which is not DF)

4 tablespoons of chopped fresh coriander (cilantro) and mint leaves

1 small red chilli, seeded and finely chopped

Salt and freshly ground black pepper

LAMB DAUPHINOISE

750g/26oz/3⅓ cups of best lean minced lamb

4 plump cloves of garlic, peeled and crushed

1 onion, peeled and chopped

Salt, freshly ground black pepper and grated nutmeg

1 tablespoon of dried mixed herbs

1 tablespoon of tomato purée (paste)

300ml/10fl oz/1¼ cups of red wine

1 tablespoon (GF) cornflour (cornstarch)

1 large or 2 small celeriac, peeled

30g/1oz/2 tablespoons of (DF) margarine

Cayenne pepper

Preheat the oven to 200°C/400°F/Gas mark 6

First make the sauce. Mix all of the ingredients together, cover and chill until needed. Cook the mince for a few minutes in a large pan over a low heat until it is evenly browned. Stir occasionally and do not allow it to stick. Add three quarters of the garlic and the onion and cook for 2 minutes, stirring all the time. Add the seasoning, mixed herbs and tomato purée (paste). Mix in the wine and simmer for 3 minutes.

Blend the cornflour (cornstarch) with 300ml/10fl oz/1¼ cups of cold water in a mug until it is smooth. Stir the mixture into the lamb. Now bring the mince to the boil so that it thickens. Transfer this to a deep heatproof baking dish.

Remove any blemishes from the celeriac and chop it into thin and even slices, so it looks like potato slices. Have a saucepan of boiling water ready and blanch the prepared celeriac for 5 minutes. Drain and refresh under cold water.

Arrange a layer of celeriac over the mince, dot with margarine, the remaining garlic, salt and pepper. Cover with another layer of celeriac until it is all used up. Sprinkle the top with a little cayenne pepper and dot with more margarine. Bake until the celeriac is soft and cooked through, and the top is golden brown, about 45 minutes. Now reduce the heat to 180°C/350°F/Gas mark 4 and cook for another 40 minutes.

Serve hot with a dollop of the sauce on the celeriac. Ideal with a green or mixed salad.

Orange Stuffed Lamb

Keep the lamb bones to make stock if you have time. Cool and refrigerate the drained stock, skim off the set fat and discard. Use the fresh stock (bouillon) in your recipe.

Serves 8

WF DF

Thickly grated rind and juice of 1 large orange

1 tablespoon of chopped fresh mixed herbs

2 plump cloves of garlic, peeled and crushed

300ml/10fl oz/1¼ cups of water and white wine, mixed

2.2kg/4lb 12oz leg of lamb (weighed with bone and then boned and butterflied by your butcher)

Grated rind of 1 orange

15g/½oz/1 tablespoon of (DF) margarine

85g/3oz/1½ cups of 100% (WF) rye breadcrumbs

300ml/10fl oz/1¼ cups of (WF) lamb stock (bouillon)

100g/3½oz/½ cup of dried apricots, finely chopped

30g /1oz/1¼ cup of pine nuts

1 large orange, segmented and chopped

3 heaped tablespoons of finely chopped fresh parsley

Sea salt and freshly ground black pepper

1 heaped tablespoon of (GF) cornflour (cornstarch), mixed with a little cold water

Preheat the oven to 190°C/375°F/Gas mark 5

Put the grated orange rind and juice in a roasting tin with half the mixed herbs and one of the cloves of crushed garlic.

Pour over the water and wine mixture.

Next stuff the lamb. In a large bowl, mix together the grated rind of 1 orange, the remaining herbs and crushed garlic, mash in the margarine, breadcrumbs, 3 tablespoons of stock (bouillon), apricots, nuts, chopped orange, parsley and seasoning. Fill the lamb cavity with this mixture and then tie up at 25mm/1 inch intervals, using a skewer to fasten the end and keep in the stuffing. Place in the pan and pour over all the remaining stock (bouillon). Roast for 1½ hours, until crispy on the outside and pink inside. Leave to sit for 10 minutes before transferring to a carving board. Make the gravy by boiling up the juices in the pan and scraping them around. Stir in the cornflour (cornstarch) and bring to the boil until thick and clear. Serve with the carved lamb.

Lamb Fillet with Black Bean Salsa

I have used this recipe for black bean salsa with several other dishes, as familiarity makes for speed and ease in the kitchen.

Serves 6

1 quantity of Black Bean Salsa (see *page 91*)
4 large boneless lamb neck fillets, trimmed
Chilli olive oil

Salt and freshly ground black pepper
1 tablespoon of fresh coriander (cilantro) leaves

First make the salsa and chill until needed.
When you are nearly ready to serve the meat, brush the lamb with a little chilli olive oil and season with salt and pepper. Grill (broil) or fry until crispy on the outside and pink inside (or according to taste), about 5–7 minutes on each side.
Carve the meat, arrange the slices on warm plates with a spoonful of the salsa beside it and decorate with a few coriander (cilantro) leaves.
Serve the remaining salsa separately.
Delicious with new potatoes and a green salad.

Low-fat Oriental Pork

A number of Chinese dishes contain monosodium glutamate, which has wheat in it. Unfortunately, this makes it a no-no for Coeliacs and prevents them being able to enjoy their local Chinese take-away. This recipe has no MSG and as it doesn't use any oil, it is also an excellent low-fat dish if you feel like a Chinese-style treat!

Serves 4

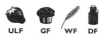

ULF GF WF DF

1 red onion, peeled and finely chopped

300ml/10fl oz/1¼ cups of water

300ml/10fl oz/1¼ cups of (GF) vegetable stock (bouillon)

300ml/10fl oz/1¼ cups of unsweetened pineapple juice

Salt and freshly ground black pepper

2 tablespoons of tomato ketchup

2 small carrots, peeled and cut into matchsticks

1 red pepper, cored and thinly sliced

1 yellow pepper, cored and thinly sliced

1 mild or hot red chilli, seeded and thinly sliced

2 cloves of garlic, peeled and crushed

1 tablespoon of grated root ginger

400g/14oz/2 generous cups of stir-fry lean pork pieces, all visible fat removed

285g/10oz of mangetouts (snowpeas), trimmed

2 tablespoons of (GF) dark soy sauce

1 tablespoon of (GF) cornflour (cornstarch)

1 tablespoon of wine vinegar

Chopped fresh coriander (cilantro) leaves to decorate

Put the onion and water in a non-stick frying pan (skillet) or wok, and bring to the boil over high heat. Cook the onion until the water has evaporated, then add the stock (bouillon) and pineapple juice. Season with salt and pepper, stir in the ketchup and add the carrots, peppers, chilli, garlic and root ginger. Cook for 5 minutes, then add the pork, mangetouts (snowpeas) and soy sauce. Cook for 3–4 minutes, stirring the ingredients frequently to make sure that they are evenly cooked and coated with the sauce.

Mix the cornflour (cornstarch) and vinegar together. Stir this into the mixture and cook until the sauce is thick, clear and coating all the ingredients.

Sprinkle with chopped fresh coriander (cilantro) leaves and serve immediately with boiled rice or boiled rice noodles.

Pork Chops with Lemon and Walnut Fettuccini

The lemon juice cuts through the richness of the pork making this a light meal. You can use veal escalopes for an even lighter dish.

Serves 4

6–12 pork chops, trimmed of fat and boned
1 tablespoon of chilli olive oil
Salt and freshly ground black pepper
12 fresh sage leaves
2 plump cloves of garlic, peeled and crushed
1 teaspoon of ground cloves
500g/17oz/6 cups of corn and parsley (GF) fettuccini

Extra oil (either sunflower, olive or chilli oil)
200ml/7fl oz/³/₄ cup of white wine
The juice of 6 small lemons
The grated rind of 2 lemons
100g/3¹/₂oz/1 cup of chopped walnuts
2 tablespoons of finely chopped parsley

Using a large pan, fry the chops over a medium heat in the chilli olive oil, seasoning them with salt, pepper and sage leaves.

Turn them over, add the garlic and cloves, reduce the heat and simmer until cooked through.

Cook the pasta in salted, boiling water in a large saucepan. Drain and refresh under hot water. Return to the pan, toss in the extra oil of your choice and cover the pan.

Add the wine and then the lemon juice, rind, and the walnuts to the pork chops and adjust the seasoning to taste. Cook for a few minutes, so that the flavours mellow.

Serve the pasta in a large shallow dish and arrange the chops over it.

Spoon over all the sauce, sprinkle with parsley and serve immediately.

CHAPTER 6

Poultry and Game

Chicken in Walnut and Garlic Sauce

European walnuts are sweeter and milder than Californian nuts, and are very compatible with pasta or as an extra source of protein. This easy and unusual dish can be served with rice and a salad.

Serves 8

8 large chicken breasts, off the bone

12 tablespoons of olive oil

6 heaped tablespoons of roughly chopped walnuts

6 heaped tablespoons of chopped parsley

6 plump cloves of garlic, peeled and crushed

Plenty of salt and freshly ground black pepper

Preheat the oven to 200°C/400°F/Gas mark 6

Place the chicken breasts in an ovenproof serving dish.

Put all the remaining ingredients into a food processor and whiz briefly into a sauce.

Spread the mixture over the chicken and bake in the oven for 40 minutes until golden and cooked through.

Serve hot with potatoes, rice, pasta or bread to soak up all the lovely juices.

Baked Chicken and Spinach Crumble

A cheap and cheerful kitchen lunch or supper party dish, ideal for both children and adults. It is perfect with baked potatoes.

Serves 6

6 chicken leg/thigh pieces, or 1 whole chicken cut into 6 portions	3 heaped tablespoons of oats
1 tablespoon of (GF) vegetable stock (bouillon) powder in 500ml/17fl oz/2 cups of water	1 tablespoon of fresh thyme leaves
1 sprig of rosemary	500g/17oz/9 cups of frozen leaf spinach, defrosted
1 bay leaf	1 heaped tablespoon of (DF) margarine plus 1 heaped teaspoon
1 plump clove of garlic, peeled and crushed	2 tablespoons of (GF) cornflour (cornstarch)
Salt and freshly ground black pepper and grated nutmeg	240ml/8fl oz/1 cup of soya cream
4 thick slices of 100% pure rye-bread, processed into breadcrumbs	A little cayenne pepper
	Sunflower oil

Preheat the oven to 200°C/400°F/Gas mark 6

Place the chicken pieces in a deep ovenproof dish, add the stock (bouillon), water, rosemary, bay leaf, garlic, salt, pepper and nutmeg, and cook until tender – about 40 minutes. Cover with foil to keep the meat moist.

Meanwhile, mix the breadcrumbs, oats and thyme together with just a little salt, pepper and nutmeg. Cook the spinach for a few minutes in boiling water and drain. Dot with margarine and season to taste with a little salt, pepper and nutmeg and keep covered.

Drain all the juices from the chicken dish into a bowl and arrange the chicken neatly again. Make a white sauce in a saucepan by melting 1 heaped tablespoon of margarine and stirring in the cornflour (cornstarch). Gradually incorporate all the stock (bouillon) and juices until you have a thick smooth sauce. Stir in the soya cream and adjust seasoning.

Spoon this sauce all over the chicken and then cover with spinach and top with all the crumble mixture. Sprinkle with a little cayenne pepper and sunflower oil and bake for 30 minutes until golden and bubbling.

Prune and Walnut Stuffed Roast Chicken

A wonderful wintery combination that is also delicious stuffed into pheasant or turkey.

Serves 6

1 onion, finely chopped

2 tablespoons of olive oil

1 plump clove of garlic, peeled and crushed

55g/2oz/½ cup of walnut pieces, finely chopped

255g/9oz/1¼ cups of chopped, ready-to-eat stoned (pitted) prunes

Salt and freshly ground black pepper

½ teaspoon of (GF) mixed (pie) spice

2 tablespoons of dry sherry

1 beaten egg

55g/2oz/⅔ cup of ground almonds

2 bay leaves

1.9kg/4.2lb free-range roasting chicken

9 rashers of rindless streaky bacon

4 sprigs of thyme

200ml/7fl oz/¾ cup of dry cider

½ a (GF) chicken stock cube dissolved in 200ml/ 7fl oz/¾ cup of boiling water

1 tablespoon of (GF) cornflour (cornstarch), dissolved in 1 tablespoon of cold water

2 tablespoons of chopped fresh parsley

In a non-stick pan, fry the onion in the oil until soft, for about 5 minutes, then add the garlic, walnuts, prunes, salt, pepper and mixed (pie) spice.

Cook for a couple of minutes and then add the sherry. As soon as it has evaporated, remove the saucepan from the heat and stir in the beaten egg and ground almonds.

Grease a large ovenproof dish with a little oil. Lay a bay leaf at each end.

Remove the fat pockets from the inside of the chicken and then slide a sharp knife under the breast skin and all over the meat. This is where you will put the stuffing. Insert a level tablespoon of stuffing into this area and pack the skin down into a good shape.

Now wrap the bacon strips around the chicken breast and squeeze gently into a neat packet.

Place in the dish on the bay leaves and sprinkle with the thyme and more salt and pepper.

Mix the cider with the stock and water mixture and pour around the chicken. Bake for 1–1¼ hours until the bacon is crispy and the chicken has cooked through (if the bacon gets too crispy, cover it loosely with foil). The chicken is ready when the juices run clear when tested with a skewer.

Place the chicken on a warm plate while you transfer the juices to a small saucepan.

Stir in the cornflour (cornstarch) and bring to the boil until cooked, thickened and clear again.

Serve slices of chicken on a warm plate with a pool of sauce and sprinkle over a little chopped fresh parsley.

Turkey Loaf with Bean and Lime Salsa

Broad (fava) beans are full of vitamin C, iron and fibre. Choose the youngest and greenest beans for the sweetest flavour and do not over-cook or they will discolour and wrinkle.

Serves 6

ULF GF WF DF

LOAF
2–3 large courgettes (zucchini)

1 onion, peeled and finely chopped

2 large garlic cloves, peeled and crushed

900g/2lbs/4 cups of lean turkey, minced (ground)

2 heaped tablespoons of chopped fresh parsley

2 heaped tablespoons of chopped fresh chives

1 tablespoon of chopped fresh rosemary

1 large free-range egg white, lightly beaten

Salt and freshly ground black pepper

SALSA
455g/1lb/3 cups of frozen baby broad (fava) beans

1 tablespoon of dark brown sugar

425g/15oz can of peeled and chopped tomatoes

1 red chilli, seeded and finely chopped

1/2 a red onion, peeled and finely chopped

Zest and juice of 1 fresh lime

A large handful of fresh basil leaves, torn into small
  pieces

A large handful of fresh parsley leaves, finely chopped

30cm/12 inch non-stick terrine tin, lined with baking
  parchment (wax paper)

Preheat the oven to 190°C/375°F/Gas mark 5

Trim the courgettes (zucchini) and cut them into thin ribbons using a vegetable peeler or a hand-held metal cheese slicer. Bring a saucepan of water to the boil, add the courgettes (zucchini) and blanch over high heat for 1 minute. Drain and rinse under cold water.

Line the prepared tin with the courgettes (zucchini), going from side to side and ensuring that they touch each other. Cover the ends of the terrine tin with some more slices, making sure that they overlap enough to prevent gaps.

Put the onion, garlic and minced (ground) turkey in a bowl with all the herbs and beaten egg white and combine it thoroughly. Season with salt and pepper.

Place half the turkey mixture into the prepared base of the tin and level it off. Cover the mixture with any leftover courgette (zucchini) slices.

Now cover the courgettes (zucchini) with the remaining turkey mixture. Press it all firmly down and then cover with a very thick layer of baking parchment (wax paper).

Set the terrine tin in a baking tray with enough water to come one third of the way up the side of the terrine tin.

Place the tray in the oven and bake for 1 1/2 hours or until the loaf is cooked through. (The terrine is ready when an inserted skewer comes out clean and the juices are clear.)

Meanwhile, make the salsa. Cook the broad (fava) beans in boiling water for about 5 minutes or until tender. Drain them and refresh under cold water. When the beans are cool enough to touch, peel off the skins and discard them.

Put the beans into a bowl, mix in all the remaining salsa ingredients and season to taste. Chill the mixture until the turkey loaf is ready.

When the turkey loaf is cooked through, cool slightly so that you can remove the paper and turn it out onto a serving dish. Peel off the remaining paper and serve the loaf hot with the chilled bean and lime salsa.

Turkey Breasts in Sage and Polenta Crumbs

I use lots of turkey now that it is so easy to buy ready-sliced into escalopes.

Serves 4

4 thick turkey escalopes, trimmed of all fat

4 thick slices of hard goat's or sheep's cheese

20 large sage leaves

6 slices of Parma ham (prosciutto), fat trimmed off

2 tablespoons of rice flour

Salt and freshly ground black pepper

2 eggs, beaten

4 tablespoons of polenta (maize) crumbs

Sunflower oil, to fry

Slice each escalope in half horizontally and lay out open. Place a slice of cheese and 3 sage leaves in each escalope and wrap 1½ pieces of Parma ham (prosciutto) around each fillet (to secure). Season the flour with salt and pepper and then dust each escalope with it. Dip the escalopes in the beaten eggs and then roll in a plate of polenta crumbs. Heat the oil in a frying pan (skillet), add the remaining sage and fry the escalopes on each side for 5–6 minutes until crispy golden brown and cooked through. Drain on kitchen (paper) towels and serve immediately with new potatoes and salad.

Chestnut Stuffed Turkey with Bread Sauce and Cranberry Sauce

Christmas is always a difficult time for people with allergies, so there are plenty of Christmas and New Year recipes in this book for everyone to enjoy. Buy (GF) sausages in advance and freeze them so that you can have them with traditional bacon rolls.

Serves 6–8

4kg/8.8lb large free-range turkey with giblets
1 onion, peeled and sliced
Plenty of fresh thyme and 3 bay leaves
2 whole cloves
Salt and freshly ground black pepper

STUFFING
455g/16oz/2 cups of raw (GF) sausage meat
425g/15oz/2 cups of chickpeas (garbanzo beans)
180ml/6fl oz/³/₄ cup of sunflower oil
6 tablespoons of dry sherry
225g/8oz/1¹/₂ cups of prepared whole chestnuts,
   roughly chopped
Grated nutmeg
1 heaped teaspoon of allspice
1 heaped teaspoon of (GF) mixed (pie) spice
130g/4¹/₂oz/1 cup of luxury dried mixed fruit
1 large free-range egg, beaten
8 slices of smoked streaky bacon

200ml/7fl oz/³/₄ cup of dry white wine or
   unsweetened apple juice
Oil for brushing
1 tablespoon of (GF) cornflour (cornstarch) dissolved
   in 2 tablespoons of water

BREAD SAUCE
100g/3¹/₂oz/²/₃ cup of flaked or ground white rice
200ml/7fl oz/³/₄ cup of coconut milk
200ml/7fl oz/³/₄ cup of soya cream
1 heaped teaspoon of (DF) margarine

CRANBERRY SAUCE
680g/24oz of fresh or frozen cranberries
The grated rind and juice of 2 oranges
4 tablespoons of sugar
A little (GF) cornflour (cornstarch) and cold water,
   mixed (optional)

Preheat the oven to 190°C/375°F/Gas mark 5

Pull out any fat from inside the turkey and discard.

Put the giblets along with half the onion, some thyme, 1 bay leaf, 2 cloves, salt and pepper in a deep pan and cover with 2 litres/70fl oz/2 quarts of water. Bring to the boil, then simmer for 2 hours until you have a good stock, topping up with water half way through if necessary (to make sure you end up with 1 litre/35fl oz/4 cups). Drain the stock into a bowl and keep cool until needed.

Next prepare the stuffing. Mix the sausage meat and chickpeas (garbanzo beans), oil and sherry in a food processor and process until smooth. Scrape this mixture into a large bowl and mix in the chestnuts, which will break them up a little more. Season with salt and pepper. Add some grated

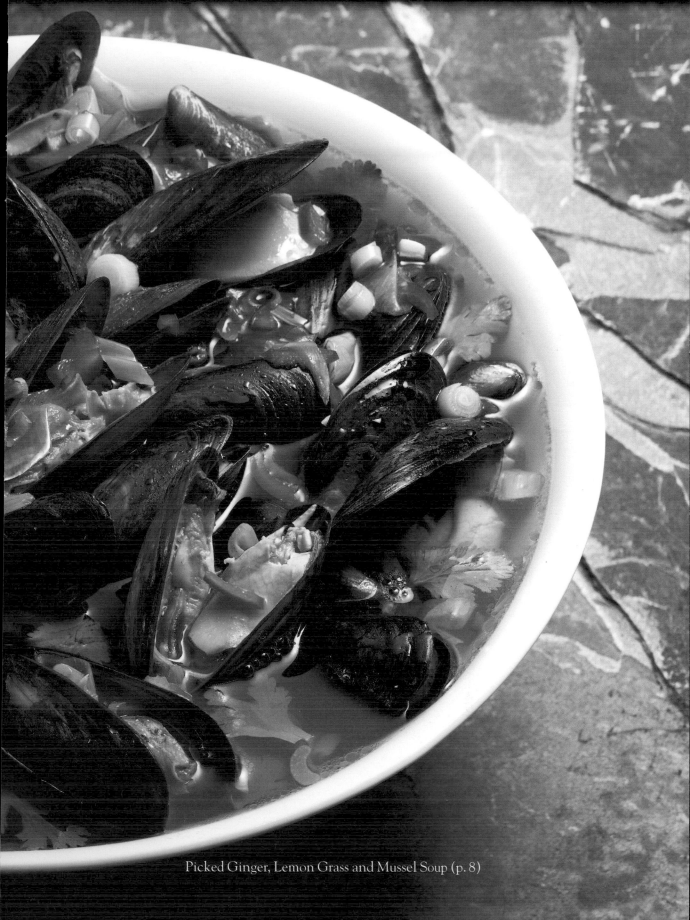

Picked Ginger, Lemon Grass and Mussel Soup (p. 8)

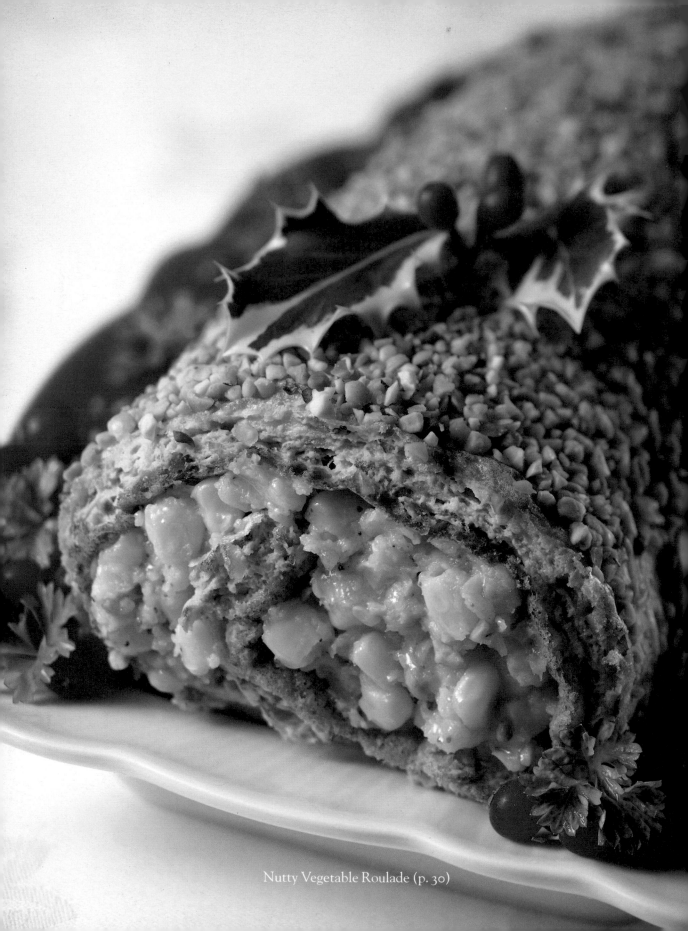

Nutty Vegetable Roulade (p. 30)

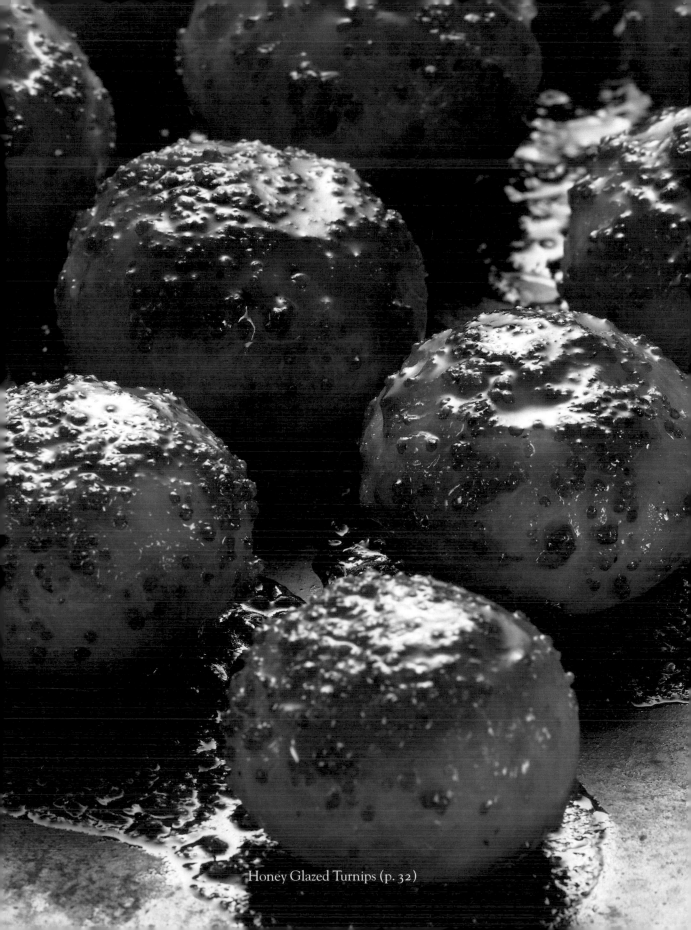
Honey Glazed Turnips (p. 32)

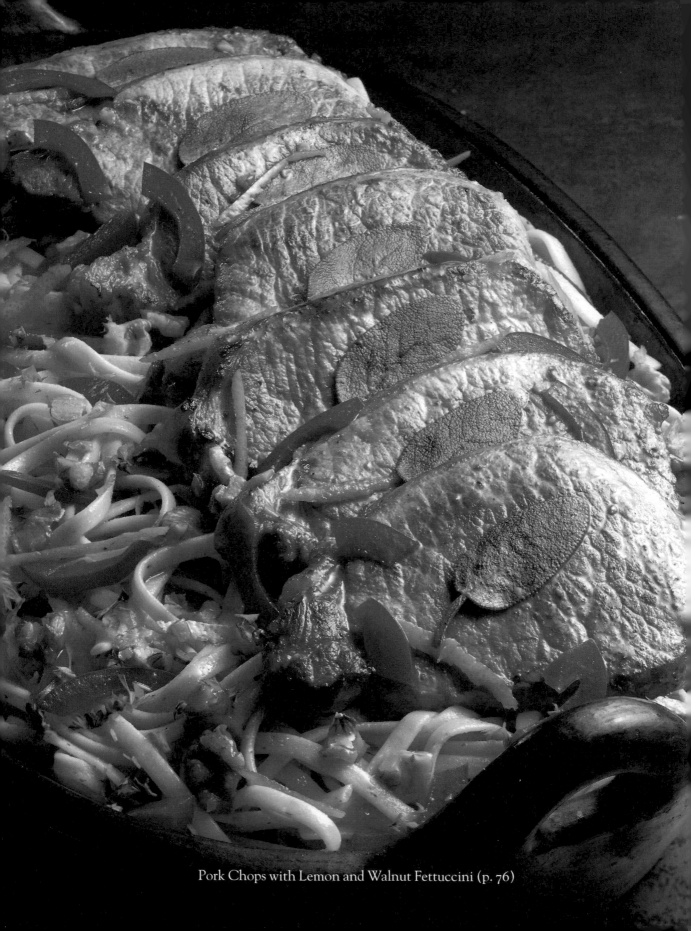

Pork Chops with Lemon and Walnut Fettuccini (p. 76)

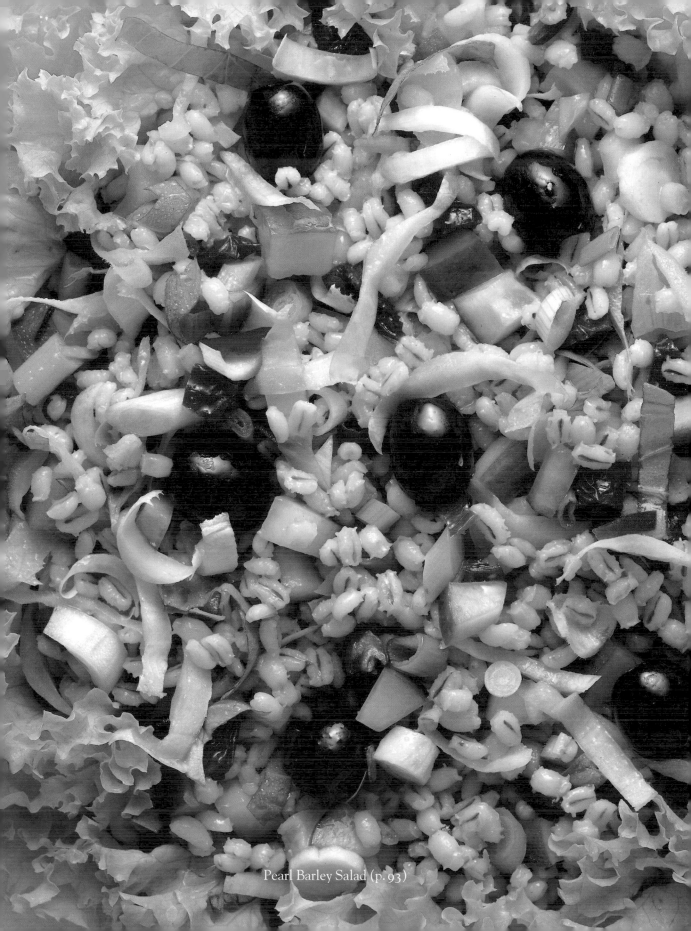

Pearl Barley Salad (p. 93)

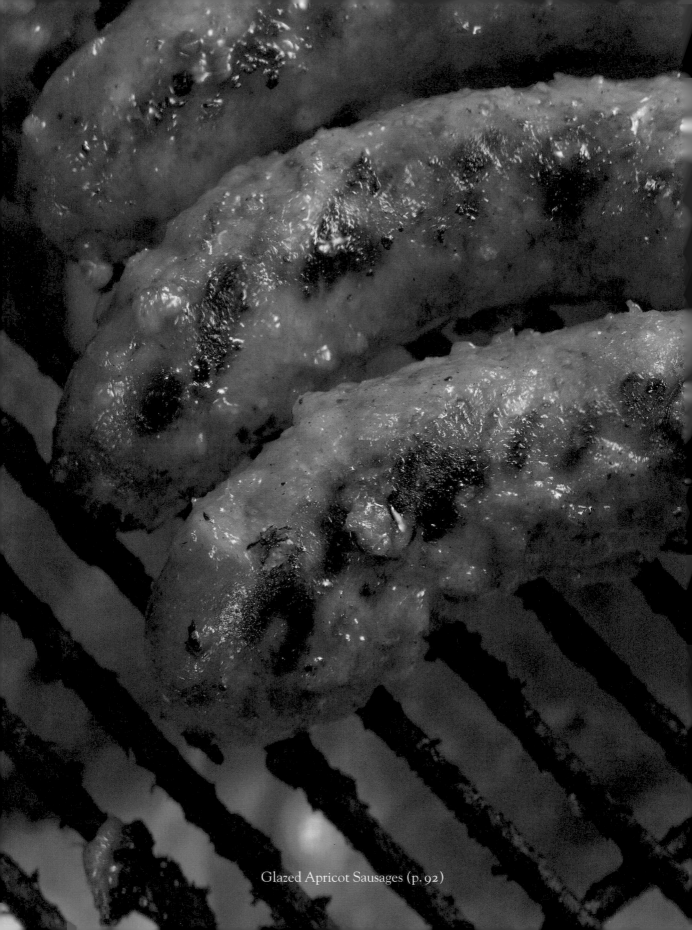

Glazed Apricot Sausages (p. 92)

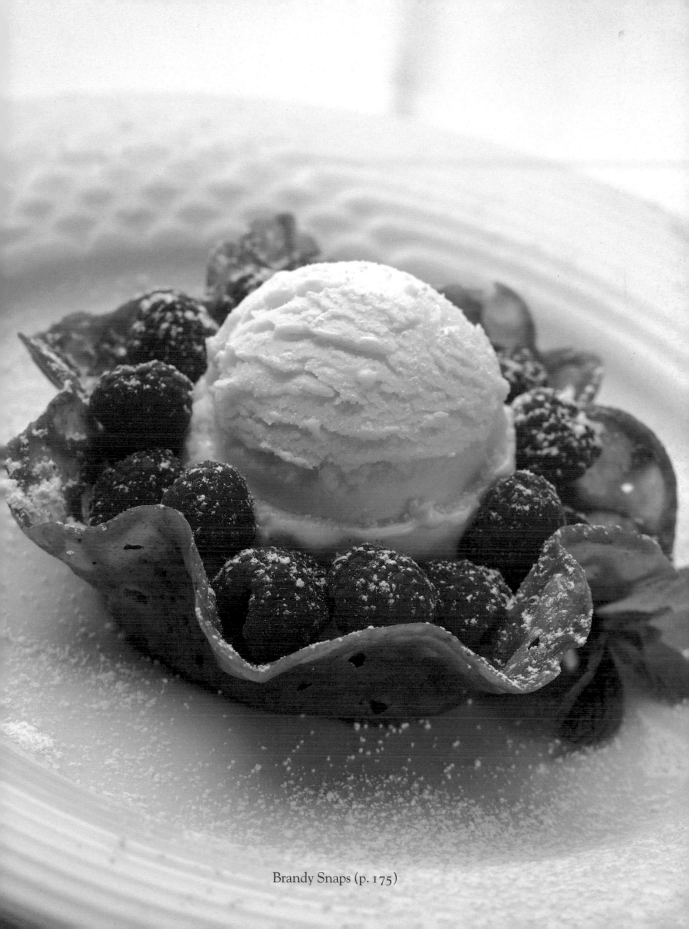

Brandy Snaps (p. 175)

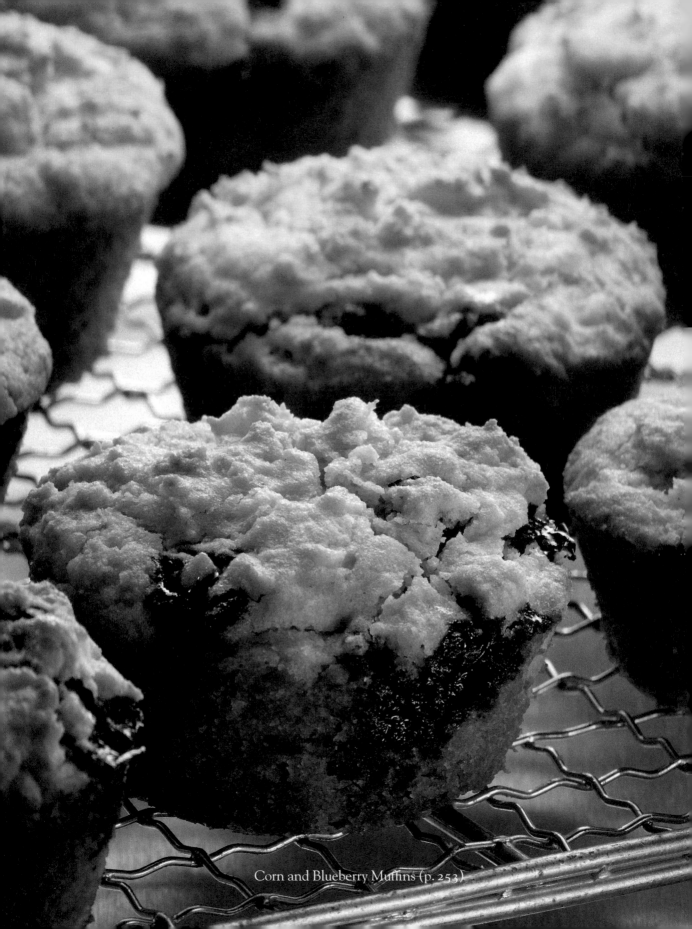

Corn and Blueberry Muffins (p. 253)

nutmeg, allspice, mixed (pie) spice and fresh thyme to taste. Then add the dried fruit and the beaten egg and mix well.

Carefully lift the skin up from the whole turkey breast and bone with a sharp knife, taking care not to break the skin. Carefully push the stuffing up under the skin as far as you can until it is packed full. Shape it roundly with your clean hands and then wrap up in bacon.

Put the turkey in a roasting tin on a bed of the remaining onion, bay leaves, some thyme, salt, pepper and wine or juice. Brush the turkey all over with oil and a little more salt, pepper and thyme.

Cover with foil and roast the turkey for 2 hours, topping up the liquid level with stock. Remove the foil from the turkey and roast for another 30 minutes until golden. When the legs are pierced, the juices should run clear. Let the turkey sit for 15 minutes before carving.

Meanwhile, make the gravy. Drain off all the juices into a pan, discard the onions and bay leaves, and remove the excess fat with a spoon. Add enough of the remaining stock to make lots of gravy. Stir in the cornflour (cornstarch) dissolved in cold water. Bring to the boil and cook for a few minutes. Adjust the seasoning and transfer to sauce boats.

To make the bread sauce, put the rice, coconut milk, salt, pepper and freshly grated nutmeg into a non-stick saucepan and simmer until soft and creamy. Add the soya cream and margarine, and keep warm until needed.

To make the cranberry sauce, mix all of the ingredients and simmer for 10 minutes until the cranberries have burst and are soft and pulping. If the sauce is too runny, stir in extra cornflour (cornstarch) and water mixed together and bring to the boil until it is clear and thick.

Serve the turkey and sauces with (GF) sausages, bacon rolls, roast potatoes, Brussels sprouts and chestnuts.

Duck with Thyme and Bacon

This duck dish is robust, wintery and more filling with lots of beans. A good way of using up the legs nobody ate.

Serves 2

4 small or 2 large duck legs, raw or cooked

A little olive oil

1 teaspoon of fresh thyme leaves

Salt and freshly ground black pepper

1 red onion, peeled and finely sliced into rings

2 tablespoons of olive oil

6 smoked rindless bacon rashers, chopped

1 clove of garlic, peeled and crushed

455g/16oz/2 1/2 cups of canned borlotti beans, drained

1 bay leaf

1 sprig of fresh thyme

200ml/7fl oz/3/4 cup of (GF) chicken stock (bouillon)

200ml/7fl oz/3/4 cup of dry white wine

A little fresh basil to decorate

Rub the raw legs with a little olive oil, 1 teaspoon of fresh thyme leaves, and salt and pepper. Place half the onion on a roasting tray, place the legs on top and roast for 40 minutes until crispy and cooked through.

If using cooked duck, gently cook the onion first in half the oil and when cooked through, add the legs and brush with a little more oil, salt and pepper and cook for 20 minutes until hot and crispy again.

Meanwhile, sauté the rest of the onion in a saucepan with the oil, bacon and garlic until golden. Add the borlotti beans, bay leaf and sprig of thyme, season to taste and pour over the stock (bouillon) and wine. Simmer for 20 minutes, stirring from time to time.

Spoon the beans and sauce onto a hot plate and place the legs on top. Sprinkle with a little shredded basil and serve with a crispy green salad.

Venison Loaf and Red Pepper Sauce

This is brilliant for a picnic as well as for a kitchen supper. (GF) breads, salad and a good (GF) chutney are all that is needed.

Serves 5

2 tablespoons of olive oil	SAUCE
1 onion, peeled and finely chopped	1 onion, peeled and chopped
455g/16oz/2 cups of raw minced venison	1 tablespoon of olive oil
455g/16oz/2 cups of raw (GF) sausage meat	2 large red peppers, cored, seeded and chopped
1 tablespoon of chopped fresh tarragon leaves	2 cloves of garlic, peeled and crushed
1 teaspoon of chopped fresh parsley	2 chillies, seeded and chopped
2 plump cloves of garlic, peeled and crushed	1 teaspoon of thyme leaves
Salt, pepper and grated nutmeg	500ml/17fl oz/2 cups of carrot juice
1 teaspoon of allspice	Salt and freshly ground black pepper
1 large free-range egg, beaten	
1 tablespoon of (GF) Worcestershire sauce	A non-stick metal terrine/loaf tin
A little (GF) chilli sauce/oil	

Preheat the oven to 200°C/400°F/Gas mark 6

Heat the oil in a pan, add the onions and cook until soft but not brown, about 10 minutes.
Put the onions into a large bowl and mix in all the remaining ingredients.
Fill the tin with the venison mixture. Pat down firmly, cover with foil brushed with oil and bake in a shallow tray of water for 1 hour or until the juices run clear when a skewer is inserted.
Leave the loaf for 15 minutes before turning it out onto a serving plate, either to eat hot with the sauce or cover and chill until needed.
To make the sauce, cook the onion in the oil with the peppers, garlic, chillies and thyme for 5 minutes over a medium heat. Add the carrot juice and season. Cook for 25 minutes over a moderate heat and stir to prevent sticking. Allow to cool and then liquidize. Adjust the seasoning and reheat to serve with the venison loaf.

Venison and Pickled Walnut Casserole

I always imagined that pickled walnuts were sweet and boozy, so I was very surprised when I was actually brave enough to taste one and discovered it wasn't remotely how I imagined, and rather delicious in this recipe.

Serves 6–8

WF   DF

2 tablespoons of olive oil

3 onions, peeled and finely sliced

1.2kg/2lb 11oz/5½ cups of stewing venison cubes

130g/4½oz/¾ cup of streaky bacon with rinds removed, chopped

2 heaped tablespoons of brown sugar

2 cloves of garlic, peeled and crushed

1 bay leaf

A small bunch of fresh thyme

2 sprigs of rosemary, leaves only

1 tablespoon of (GF) Worcestershire sauce

2 heaped tablespoons of tomato purée (paste)

Salt and freshly ground black pepper to taste

500ml/17fl oz/2 cups of red wine

790g/27oz/9 cups of pickled walnuts in malt vinegar

2 tablespoons of (GF) cornflour (cornstarch), dissolved in 3 tablespoons of cold water

30g/1oz/2 tablespoons of (DF) margarine

Preheat the oven to 180°C/350°F/Gas mark 4

Put the oil in a casserole dish and slowly cook the onions for 8 minutes on the top of the stove. Then turn up the heat and sauté the venison cubes with the onions for a further 8 minutes. Now stir in the bacon, sugar, garlic, herbs, Worcestershire sauce, tomato purée (paste), salt and pepper. Pour in the wine and cover. Leave to simmer for 35 minutes.

Halve the walnuts before adding them with a tablespoon of the vinegar. (Throw out the remainder of the vinegar.)

Transfer the venison casserole to the hot oven, cook for 1 hour and then turn the oven off and leave to cool.

Before serving, place the casserole back on top of the stove and reheat. Add the dissolved cornflour (cornstarch) to the casserole and cook slowly until thickened. Cut the margarine into pieces and stir into the sauce to glaze. Adjust the seasoning if necessary and serve with the Sweet Potato and Orange Purée (*see page 35*) or Exotic Pea Purée (*see page 29*).

CHAPTER 7

Buffets, Barbecues and Picnics

Chicken in Red Pesto Sauce

A couple of jars of this and that and you have a bright and colourful alternative to the inevitable coronation chicken.

Serves 12

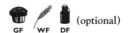

370g/13oz/1½ cups of sun-dried tomato purée or paste
100g/3½oz/¾ cup of pine nuts
100g/3½oz/¾ cup of grated sheep's or goat's hard cheese (if you can eat it, omit this if not)
2 whole extra large cooked chickens
600g/21oz/2⅓ cups of (DF/GF) mayonnaise

800ml/28fl oz/3⅓ cups of coconut cream
Salt and freshly ground black pepper
(GF) chilli sauce/oil to taste
90ml/3fl oz/⅓ cup of cold water
4 mild red chillies, left whole for decoration
Fresh parsley, basil or coriander (cilantro) to decorate

Put the tomato paste and pine nuts into the food processor and blend. Add the grated sheep's or goat's cheese to taste (if being used).

Strip both the chickens of their meat and discard the bones and skins. Chop the meat into bite size pieces. Put the meat into a large bowl with the mayonnaise, red pesto sauce, and coconut cream, and mix well. Season to taste with salt, pepper and chilli sauce/oil. Add the water to loosen the mixture to a perfect consistency.

Tip the mixture into a serving dish and decorate with chillies and herbs. Serve with Wild Rice and Water Chestnut Salad or Pearl Barley Salad (*see pages 95 and 93*).

Turkey Burgers and Black Bean Salsa

With all the beef food scares, turkey has become one of the new safe foods. The same ground rules apply: do not burn the outside, leaving the inside raw; cook slowly all the way through; don't leave the raw burgers near or in the heat, and keep chilled until needed.

This is a good low-fat option, and is delicious with any sort of salsa or barbecue sauce.

Serves 6–8 or

6 ready-made (GF) or (WF) beefburger buns or Corn
   Meal Pancakes (*see page 24*)
900g/32oz/4 cups of minced (ground) fresh turkey

MARINADE
1 red chilli, seeded and chopped
6 trimmed spring onions (scallions), finely sliced
2 cloves of garlic, peeled and crushed
2 teaspoons of ground cumin
2 teaspoons of fresh oregano
1 teaspoon of fresh thyme
1/2 teaspoon of paprika
Salt and freshly ground black pepper
The juice of 1/2 a lemon

BLACK BEAN SALSA
1 small ripe fresh mango, peeled and flesh cubed
3 spring onions (scallions), trimmed and sliced
1 clove of garlic, peeled and crushed
1/2 chilli, seeded and chopped
2 tablespoons of chopped coriander (cilantro) leaves
1 ripe tomato, skinned, seeded and chopped
The grated rind and juice of 2 limes
Salt and freshly ground black pepper
3 tablespoons of black beans (soak in water
   overnight, then boil in clean water for about 80
   minutes until tender, drain and refresh under
   cold running water)
1 ripe avocado, peeled and chopped into the juice
   of 1 lime

Mix all the marinade ingredients together in a bowl, add the turkey and marinate for a few hours. Next make the salsa. Place the mango, spring onions (scallions), garlic and chilli with the coriander (cilantro), tomato, lime zest and juice, salt and pepper in a food processor and mix for a second, just to bring it together.

Transfer to a clean bowl. Add the beans and the chopped avocado in lime juice and cover with clingfilm (plastic wrap). Chill until needed.

Now, with clean hands, divide the turkey mixture into 6 portions and shape firmly into burgers. Place on the barbecue, or char-grill in a pan until crispy and well cooked. Serve on the bun with the salsa on top or beside it.

Glazed Apricot Sausages

Venison sausages are lower in cholesterol and fat than beef and pork so I always use them for grown-up barbecues, or bangers and mash. But this works well with any type of sausage, including vegetarian.

Serves 6–12

GF / WF / DF

240g/8oz/1 generous cup ready-to-eat dried (or canned and drained) apricots
1 teaspoon of (GF) mixed (pie) spice
1 tablespoon of (GF) Worcestershire sauce
2 teaspoons of red Thai curry paste

Salt and freshly ground black pepper
300ml/10fl oz/1¼ cups of water
12–18 (GF) venison or other sausages
1 tablespoon of olive oil

Cook the apricots with the mixed (pie) spice, Worcestershire sauce, curry paste, salt and pepper in 300ml/10fl oz/1¼ cups of water over a medium heat until soft, about 20 minutes. Add 100ml/⅓fl oz/⅓ cup of water if reducing too much in the saucepan. Remove from heat, allow to cool then process to a purée.

Place the sausages in a grill (broil)-proof tray and brush with the olive oil. Spread over the apricot mixture and marinate for up to 24 hours.

Barbecue or grill (broil) them until cooked through and crispy on the outside.

Serve with baked potatoes.

Pearl Barley Salad

This is a jolly and bright salad, ideal for all age groups and all types of parties. For a bigger party, double the ingredients for 10–12, treble them for 14–18.

Serves 6

V WF DF

200g/7oz/1 cup of pearl barley

1 tablespoon of olive oil

500ml/17fl oz/2 cups of (WF) vegetable stock (bouillon)

Pinch of saffron

The juice of 2 lemons

75ml/2½fl oz/¼ cup of olive oil

Sea salt and freshly ground black pepper

½ cucumber, peeled, seeded and cubed

4 sun-dried tomatoes, chopped

12 large black olives, stoned (pitted)

2 heads of chicory, trimmed and sliced

8 spring onions (scallions), trimmed and sliced

1 red chilli, seeded and chopped

2 tablespoons of shredded basil leaves

Sauté the barley in a pan with the tablespoon of oil for a minute and then add the vegetable stock (bouillon) and saffron. Simmer for 45 minutes, topping up with water if necessary. Drain and turn into a salad bowl.

Flavour with the lemon juice, 75ml/2½fl oz/¼ cup of olive oil and seasoning. Stir in the cucumber, tomatoes, olives, chicory, spring onions (scallions) and chilli. Sprinkle with basil leaves and serve with quiche and vegetable dishes.

Black Bean, Olive and Egg Salad

Preparations for this salad need to be started the day before, but it's so easy and has the bonus of being inexpensive. It is also vegetarian friendly.

Serves 12

255g/8oz/1½ cups of black beans, soaked overnight in cold water and left covered in a cool place

1 onion studded with 2 cloves

2 bay leaves

2 sprigs of thyme

550g/19oz/4¾ cups of courgettes (zucchini), trimmed and sliced

2 large cloves of garlic, peeled and crushed

Salt and freshly ground black pepper

500g/17oz/2½ cups of sweetcorn kernels, drained (or the equivalent of frozen and defrosted sweetcorn kernels)

6 hard boiled eggs, peeled and quartered

400g/14oz/1¾ cups of capers in vinegar, drained

200ml/7fl oz/¾ cup of cider vinegar

300ml/10fl oz/1¼ cups of olive oil

(GF) chilli sauce/oil to taste

1 tablespoon of caster (superfine) sugar

4 tablespoons chopped parsley

Drain the beans and cook them with the onion, bay leaves and thyme in salted, boiling water until soft, about 1½ hours. Drain and refresh them under cold water. Transfer the beans to a huge salad bowl, remove the onion and herbs and discard.

Briefly cook the courgettes (zucchini) in boiling water so that they are still crunchy. Refresh and drain under cold water. Add the courgettes (zucchini), garlic, salt and pepper to the beans and mix well. Leave to cool before mixing in the sweetcorn, eggs, olives and capers.

In another bowl, beat the vinegar with the oil, chilli, sugar and three quarters of the parsley. Add the dressing to the salad and mix gently. Sprinkle with the remaining parsley and serve, or chill until needed.

Wild Rice and Water Chestnut Salad

Notoriously boring rice salads always seem to be produced at parties. So I feel something a bit more original is needed to add a spark of interest to any buffet.

Serves 8

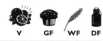

600g/21oz/3 cups of wild rice

2 mild red chillies, halved and trimmed

1 tablespoon of sesame oil

2 cloves of garlic, peeled and crushed

2 bunches of spring onions (scallions), trimmed and finely chopped

455g/16oz/2 ½ cups of water chestnuts, drained and roughly chopped

Salt and freshly ground black pepper

2 tablespoons of (GF) soy sauce

4 tablespoons of olive or sunflower oil

4 tablespoons of fresh coriander (cilantro) leaves

Cook the rice in boiling water until just soft. Drain and refresh under hot water.

Chop up the chillies finely. Heat the sesame oil in a pan, add the garlic and chilli, and heat briefly. Add the onions and the chestnuts and cook for a couple of minutes. Season with salt and pepper and soy sauce before mixing in the rice. Adjust the seasoning and stir in the oil.

Mix in half the coriander (cilantro) leaves. Cover and chill. Serve with the remaining coriander (cilantro) leaves sprinkled on top.

Spinach and Rice Torte

Serves 6

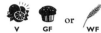

1 litre/35fl oz/4 cups of (GF) vegetable stock (bouillon)

200g/7oz/1 cup of risotto rice and a little salt

Sea salt, freshly ground black pepper and grated nutmeg

4 tablespoons of extra virgin olive oil

115g/4oz/½ cup of (DF) margarine

2 large leeks, finely sliced

4 cloves of garlic, peeled and crushed

700g/24oz/12 cups of fresh spinach, washed and coarsely chopped

5 large free-range eggs

8 tablespoons of freshly grated pecorino (romano) cheese or vegetarian cheese

1 teaspoon (DF) margarine

Cayenne pepper

25cm/10 inch spring-form cake tin, greased with (DF) margarine and coated with 4–6 tablespoons of 100% (WF) or (GF) breadcrumbs

Preheat the oven to 180°C/350°F/Gas mark 4

Place the stock (bouillon) in a large pan, bring to the boil, add the rice and cook for 20 minutes. Place in a large mixing bowl and season to taste with the salt, pepper and nutmeg.

Heat the oil and half the margarine in a pan. Add the leeks and cook until soft, then stir them into the rice. Leave the fat in the pan and cook the garlic. Add the remaining margarine and gradually add the spinach until it has wilted. Add the eggs and cheese.

Combine the rice and spinach mixture and pour into the prepared tin. Dot the surface with the teaspoon of margarine. Sprinkle with cayenne pepper.

Bake for 1 hour until golden brown and firm to touch. Cool, then turn out onto a plate. Serve at room temperature, with a crispy salad and new or baked potatoes.

CHAPTER 8

Warm Desserts

Crêpes Suzettes

This year we had the most romantic New Year's Eve in Paris. After a fabulous evening at the ballet, we strolled up the magnificent boulevards, which were full of hooting cars and joyful Parisians, until we reached our favourite restaurant. There, finally at 2am, we had the best crêpes Suzettes in Paris, or maybe that was the effect of the champagne!

Serves 6–8

CRÊPES

55g/2oz/scant ½ cup of rice flour
55g/2oz/scant ½ cup of barley flour
A pinch of salt
3 large free-range eggs
240ml/8fl oz/1 cup of soya milk (or goat's milk,
    which is not DF) mixed with 30g/1oz/2 tablespoons
    of melted (DF) margarine
Sunflower oil for frying

FILLING

115g/4oz/ ½ cup of (DF) margarine
4 heaped tablespoons of icing (confectioners') sugar
3 tablespoons of strained fresh orange juice
1 tablespoon of grated orange rind
1 tablespoon of Cointreau or orange liqueur
Extra (DF) margarine for frying
Extra caster (superfine) sugar

3 tablespoons of brandy and 3 tablespoons of
    Cointreau or orange liqueur

18cm/7 inch crêpe pan
Baking parchment (wax paper)

Make the crêpes first. Sift the flours into a bowl with the salt, make a well in the centre, break the eggs into the well and whisk them until thoroughly mixed.

Add half the milk and melted margarine in a steady stream and whisk, gradually making a smooth paste. Continue whisking as you add the remaining liquid in order to prevent lumps forming. Leave the batter to stand for 30 minutes.

Heat a little of the oil in the pan until a drop of the mixture sizzles and sets quickly.

Now ladle a tablespoon of the crêpe mixture into the pan and swirl it around so that the base of the pan is evenly coated. Cook until crispy and golden, then flip over and cook the other side. Continue until you have used up all the batter, layering each crêpe on baking parchment (wax paper) as you go.

Now make the filling by mixing the margarine and icing (confectioners') sugar together in a food processor until pale and light. Add the orange juice and rind with the liqueur and blend just long enough to become smooth.

Spread the filling over each crêpe and fold into a triangle. Heat a little margarine in a large frying pan (skillet), add the crêpes and sprinkle with caster (superfine) sugar. Pour over the brandy and Grand Marnier and set light to it. Cook until the flames go out and then serve immediately.

Spring Rolls and Passion Fruit Sauce

This is such a novel and exotic idea. Fiona, who is also a cook, and I, were perusing the two brand-new food magazines that she had just discovered. We love to discuss recipes and new ideas and eventually I concocted this recipe.

Serves 6 (2 each with a few spare ones)

V   GF   WF   DF

ROLLS

1 heaped teaspoon of ground ginger

340g/12oz/1½ cups of drained weight from a can of finely chopped pineapple flesh in natural juices

2 x 50g/2oz packages (GF) rice flour pancakes for spring rolls

Sunflower oil for frying

SAUCE

410g/14oz can of apricot halves in pineapple or natural juices

3 ripe passion fruit, halved with all the seeds scooped out

Fresh basil leaves to decorate, or exotic orchid flowers for special occasions

---

First, make the sauce by blending half the apricots and half the juice in a blender. You can use the remainder for decorating the serving plates. I slice them and add a little sprig of fresh basil, or an exotic orchid flower.

Mix the passion fruit pulp into the purée and place a spoonful of the passion fruit sauce on each decorated plate.

On another plate, mix the ginger with the chopped pineapple.

Put plenty of oil in a deep saucepan, no less than about 5cm/2 inches deep, so that you can fry the rolls four at a time.

Next, wet two clean tea towels with fresh tap water and wring them out thoroughly. Place individual pancakes flat on one tea towel and cover them with the second towel. After about a minute they will be soft and pliable.

Take a rice pancake and place it on a clean surface. Spoon a line of the pineapple across the paper, about two thirds of the way up it. Pull the top of the pancake over the filling, bring in and tuck in the sides and then roll up as tightly as you can. This will ensure that the filling can not escape and the rolls will not come undone.

Repeat until all the rolls are finished.

Now fry 4 pancakes at a time until they are crispy and golden all over and bobbing on the surface of the oil.

Drain the pancakes with a slotted spoon and let them sit on some kitchen (paper) towels on a plate in a hot oven until they are all ready – be as quick as you can so that they remain crispy.

To ensure maximum crispiness, serve and eat the rolls immediately on the prepared plates.

Amaretto Stuffed Peaches

Amaretto always brings a smile to my face, as it conjures up memories of sitting on the balcony of our hotel on the Amalfi Coast gazing at the glittering sea and moonlight, sipping a chilled glass of this almond nectar.

Serves 6

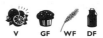

6 ripe peaches

Juice of ½ large lemon mixed with treble its quantity of cold water

Juice of 1 large orange and double its quantity of cold water

3 tablespoons of Cointreau mixed with 6 tablespoons of boiling water

55g/2oz/¾ cup of 100% rye breadcrumbs or (GF) breadcrumbs

100g/3½ oz of (GF) ratafias (dessert macaroons)

3 tablespoons of Amaretto di Saronno liqueur

Plenty of caster (superfine) sugar

Preheat the oven to 190°C/375°F/Gas mark 5

Wipe the peaches, cut them in half and remove their stones (pits).

Pour the lemon and water mixture and the orange and water mixture into a large ovenproof dish.

Neatly arrange the peaches (with the cavities facing up) in the dish and pour over the Cointreau and water mixture, ensuring some of it settles in the peach cavities.

Put the breadcrumbs, ratafias and Amaretto liqueur into a food processor and blend briefly until it forms a wet crumbly mixture.

Spoon the mixture loosely into the peach cavities.

Sprinkle the peaches with plenty of caster (superfine) sugar and bake for 45 minutes, or until the peaches are just soft but still holding their shape.

Serve the peaches warm on their own or with your choice of (DF) ice-cream or Zabaglione (*see page 119*).

Blinis with Spiced Cherries

You can play around with blinis, using them with other ingredients at other meals throughout the year. They are ideal for brunch parties, served with smoked salmon and goat's cheese. In summer, serve them with raspberries and (DF) vanilla ice-cream.

Serves 6 (2 each)

SPICED CHERRIES
30g/1oz/2 tablespoons (DF) margarine

2 x 850g/1lb 14oz cans of pitted black cherries or a jar of cherries in liqueur if you are in a real hurry!

1 teaspoon of ground cinnamon

30g/1oz/2 tablespoons of caster (superfine) sugar or to taste

Juice and zest of 1 orange

2 tablespoons of Kirsch liqueur

BLINIS
55g/2oz/generous ½ cup of buckwheat flour

55g/2oz/½ cup of rice flour

1 teaspoon of (GF) baking powder

1 teaspoon of olive oil

2 tablespoons of sunflower oil

2 medium free-range eggs, beaten

140ml/5fl oz/⅔ cup of water

A drop of extra oil for frying

(DF) vanilla ice-cream

Melt the margarine in a frying pan (skillet), add the cherries, cinnamon, sugar, orange juice and zest, and cook for a couple of minutes over medium heat. Add the Kirsch and simmer for about 5 minutes. Keep warm while you make the blinis.

Sift the flours with the baking powder into a bowl, make a well in the centre and pour in the oils and eggs. Stir with a balloon whisk and gradually incorporate the water.

Leave the batter to stand at room temperature for 15 minutes.

Heat a large, non-stick frying pan (skillet) with a drop of extra oil until very hot. Pour a spoonful of the blini mixture into the pan and repeat until you have 4 blinis, each about 6cm/2½ inch in diameter.

Cook the blinis until they are firm on the underside and bubbling on the upper side, then turn them over and cook the other side.

Keep the blinis warm until they are all ready.

Serve two of them, overlapping, on each warm plate with a pool of warm spiced cherries beside them and a scoop of (DF) vanilla ice-cream on the edge of the pancakes.

Honey and Ginger Baked Pears with Sherry Ice-cream

This is a lovely wintry combination of ginger and alcohol, which is perfect with pears. The contrast of cold ice-cream with hot pears is sublime.

Serves 6–8

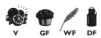

ICE-CREAM

5 large free-range egg yolks

100g/3½oz/½ cup of caster (superfine) sugar

2 teaspoons of ground ginger

4 tablespoons of ginger ale

500ml/17fl oz/2 cups of soya cream

70g/2½oz/¼ cup of stem ginger, finely chopped

4 tablespoons of pale dry sherry

PEARS

6 almost ripe pears, peeled, quartered and cored

Juice of 1 lemon

1 rounded tablespoon of caster (superfine) sugar

1 heaped teaspoon of ground ginger

55g/2oz/¼ cup of (DF) margarine

3 tablespoons of honey

4 tablespoons of ginger ale

Make the ice-cream first. Beat the egg yolks with the sugar, ginger and ginger ale in a food processor until pale and creamy. Transfer the mixture to a non-stick saucepan and blend in the soya cream and stem ginger.

Cook the custard over very low heat until it comes to the boil, stirring most of the time to make sure it doesn't go lumpy or curdle. As soon as it starts to boil, remove it from the heat.

Stir in the sherry. Leave the mixture to cool down, stirring frequently until it is cold.

As soon as the ice-cream maker is ready, churn the custard until it is frozen. Scrape the mixture into a sealable container and freeze for a few hours or until needed (this ice-cream is soft scoop and should be served directly from the freezer).

Put the prepared pears and lemon juice into a large frying pan (skillet) with the sugar, ground ginger, margarine, honey and ginger ale.

Bring the pears to the boil over medium heat and simmer for about 20 minutes, or until the pears are just soft and slightly glazed and the syrup is thick.

Serve the hot pears with the syrup on individual plates, accompanied by a large scoop of the sherry ice-cream.

Apricot Soufflé

The professional 'top hat' effect of this soufflé is created by making a circular indentation with a metal spoon in the centre of the soufflé mixture, just before cooking.

Serves 6

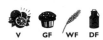

SOUFFLÉ

55g/2oz/¼ cup of (DF) margarine
30g/1oz/scant ¼ cup of (GF) cornflour (cornstarch)
3 tablespoons of orange liqueur
310ml/11fl oz/1¼ cups of the prepared apricot sauce
4 large free-range egg yolks
Zest of ½ an orange
6 large free-range egg whites
Caster (superfine) sugar and icing (confectioners')
   sugar for sprinkling

APRICOT SAUCE

255g/9oz/1¼ cups of ready-to-eat dried, stoned
   (pitted) apricots
Sugar to taste
2 tablespoons of orange liqueur
Juice from 1 orange, and zest from ½ of it

1½ litre/2 pint/3 US pint soufflé dish, greased with
   30g/1oz/2 tablespoons of (DF) margarine and
   dusted with plenty of caster (superfine) sugar

Preheat the oven to 200°C/400°F/Gas mark 6

First make the sauce. Place the apricots in a saucepan with sugar to taste and add just enough water to cover them. Simmer until soft, then purée in a blender or pass through a sieve until smooth.

Add the orange liqueur, orange zest and the juice. Add as much water as is needed to make the sauce a good pouring consistency. Measure 310ml/11fl oz/1⅓ cups of the sauce for the soufflé and transfer the rest to a serving jug, cover and keep warm until needed.

Now make the soufflé. Melt the margarine in a large saucepan over medium heat. Stir in the cornflour (cornstarch) until blended and add 3 tablespoons of orange liqueur.

Gradually stir in the measured apricot sauce until the mixture boils. Remove from the heat and beat in the egg yolks and orange zest.

In a large bowl, beat the egg whites until stiff peaks form. Using a metal spoon, fold one tablespoon of the egg whites into the apricot mixture, blending in thoroughly.

Now, quickly but gently, fold in all the remaining egg whites. Fill the prepared soufflé dish with the mixture, make an indentation in the top if you wish, and dust with caster (superfine) sugar.

Bake immediately for about 35–45 minutes, or until firm on top and golden brown. Sprinkle with sieved icing (confectioners') sugar and serve immediately with the accompanying sauce.

Hot Chocolate Soufflé

If, like me, you always have chocolate and eggs in the refrigerator, this is a wonderful emergency pudding worth its weight in gold when impromptu guests arrive!

Serves 4–6

30g/1oz/2 tablespoons of (DF) margarine

30g/1oz/scant ¼ cup of rice flour

200ml/7fl oz/¾ cup of soya milk

2 tablespoons of Cointreau or any orange liqueur

1 tablespoon of caster (superfine) sugar

140g/5oz of (DF/GF) luxury dark chocolate,
    broken up

4 large free-range egg yolks

6 egg whites

Pinch of salt

1½ litre/2 pint/3 US pint soufflé dish, greased
    with (DF) margarine and dusted with a little
    extra caster (superfine) sugar

Preheat the oven to 200°C/400°F/Gas mark 6

Melt the margarine in a saucepan. Sift in the flour and gradually beat in the milk. Bring to the boil, stirring all the time. When the sauce is thick and smooth, add the Cointreau, a tablespoon of caster (superfine) sugar and the chocolate pieces. Remove from the heat and stir until the chocolate has melted and blended with the other ingredients. Mix in the egg yolks.
Now whisk the egg whites, with a pinch of salt, in a bowl until stiff. Stir 1 spoonful of the egg whites into the chocolate mixture and then fold in the rest with a metal spoon.
Turn the mixture into the prepared soufflé dish and bake for 30 minutes until puffed, but just firm in the centre. Serve immediately.

Chocolate Pecan Pie

Pecan pie is always a success whenever it is served, so imagine the impact of a gooey chocolate one!
Serve with (DF) vanilla ice-cream for a perfect contrast.

Serves 8

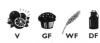

PASTRY

155g/5½oz/1 cup plus 2 tablespoons of rice flour

30g/1oz/2 tablespoons of caster (superfine) sugar

55g/2oz/⅔ cup of ground almonds

85g/3oz/6 tablespoons of (DF) margarine, cut into pieces

1 large free-range egg

2 teaspoons of lemon juice

FILLING

55g/2oz/¼ cup of (DF) margarine

3 tablespoons of (DF/GF) cocoa powder

300ml/10fl oz/1¼ cups of golden syrup (corn syrup)

3 large free-range eggs

85g/3oz/6 tablespoons of soft dark brown sugar

2 tablespoons of rum

170g/6oz/1½ cups of pecan nuts

24cm/9½ inch non-stick, loose-bottomed flan tin, greased and lined with baking parchment (wax paper)

Preheat the oven to 180°C/350°F/Gas mark 4

Place the first four pastry ingredients into a food processor and mix briefly until it resembles crumbs. Add the egg and lemon juice and process for a second or two only. Bring the mixture together using a spatula, wrap the pastry in clingfilm (plastic wrap) and chill for 2 hours.

Roll out the pastry on a floured board and then line the prepared tin with it. Prick all over the pastry base with a fork.

Make the filling by gently melting the margarine in a saucepan and stirring in the cocoa and golden syrup (corn syrup).

Beat the eggs with the brown sugar and rum in another bowl. Stir this into the syrup mixture and add the nuts.

Pour the mixture into the pie shell and bake for 40 minutes, or until the filling is just set and the pastry is golden. Serve warm.

Maple and Pumpkin Pie

A perfect pudding to serve on Guy Fawkes night or Hallowe'en. You can make it the day before and heat it up. Serve with (DF) vanilla ice-cream and all the children will be happy too.

Serves 8–12

V   GF   WF   DF

PASTRY
1 heaped tablespoon of icing (confectioners') sugar
A pinch of salt
70g/2¹/₂oz/¹/₂ cup of rice flour
70g/2¹/₂oz/¹/₂ cup of millet flour
70g/2¹/₂oz/¹/₂ cup of maize flour
140g/5oz/²/₃ cup of (DF) margarine, cut into small
   pieces
1 large free-range egg, beaten

PUDDING
200ml/7fl oz/³/₄ cup of apple juice
1 tablespoon of (GF) cornflour (cornstarch)
425g/15oz/scant 2 cups canned pumpkin
2 large free-range eggs
4 tablespoons of maple syrup
1¹/₂ teaspoons of (GF) mixed (pie) spice
1¹/₂ teaspoons of ground cinnamon
A little extra caster (superfine) sugar to sprinkle
   over the pie

23cm/9 inch non-stick, loose-bottomed pie or
   flan tin, greased

Preheat the oven to 200°C/400°F/Gas mark 6

Mix the first 5 pastry ingredients in a food processor, add the margarine and blend briefly, then add the egg to bind it all together.

Roll out the pastry and line the prepared tin. Trim off the excess pastry and keep for decorations.

Mix the apple juice and the cornflour (cornstarch) together in a small bowl. Put the pumpkin into a large bowl and stir in the apple juice mixture, followed by the eggs, maple syrup and spices. Spoon the mixture into the pastry case and level it off.

Roll out the remaining pastry, cut out pretty little decorations from it and arrange over the filling. Sprinkle the pastry on top of the pie with a little extra caster (superfine) sugar and bake the pie for about 35 minutes until the filling is firm and set and the pastry is golden brown.

Serve the pie warm.

Lime Meringue Pie

A nice change from lemon, which has become so commercialized. Serve with coconut cream as an alternative to cream, or with a (DF) vanilla ice-cream.

Serves 6

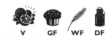

V   GF   WF   DF

115g/4oz/¹/₂ cup of (DF) margarine
100g/3 ¹/₂ oz/²/₃ cup of rice flour
70g/2 ¹/₂ oz/¹/₂ cup of maize flour
20g/³/₄ oz/1 ¹/₂ tablespoons of caster (superfine)
   sugar
1 large free-range egg yolk beaten with 2 teaspoons
   of cold water
The grated rind, pulp and juice 5 limes
The juice of 2 lemons
70g/2 ¹/₂oz/¹/₃ cup of caster (superfine) sugar
4 tablespoons of (GF) cornflour (cornstarch)
3 large free-range egg yolks
20g/³/₄oz/1 ¹/₂ tablespoons of (DF) margarine

MERINGUE
3 egg whites
170g/6oz/generous ³/₄ cup of caster (superfine) sugar

24cm/9 inch fluted non-stick flan tin
Ceramic baking balls and baking parchment
   (wax paper)

Preheat the oven to 190°C/375°F/Gas mark 5

Make the pastry by mixing the 115g/4oz/¹/₂ cup of margarine with both the flours and the 25g/³/₄oz/1 ¹/₂ tablespoons of caster (superfine) sugar in a food processor for a few seconds. Add the egg yolk and water mixture until you have a firm dough. Knead briefly on a floured board and roll out enough pastry to line the flan tin.
Bake blind with a layer of baking parchment (wax paper) and ceramic balls, until golden (about 25 minutes). Remove the balls and paper.
Meanwhile, make the filling. Put the lime rind, pulp and juice and the lemon juice into a saucepan with 60ml/2fl oz/¹/₄ cup of water and the 70g/2¹/₂oz/¹/₃ cup of sugar and heat gently until the sugar has dissolved.
Mix the cornflour (cornstarch) into a smooth paste with 5 tablespoons of cold water and then stir the mixture into the juices quickly. Now increase the heat and bring to the boil, stirring all the time. Cook for 1–2 minutes only. Cool and then beat in the 3 egg yolks and the 20g/³/₄oz/1 ¹/₂ tablespoons of margarine. Pour it into the prepared pastry.
Turn the oven heat down to 150°C/300°F/Gas mark 2.
Now make the meringue by whisking the egg whites until stiff. Now whisk in half the sugar and fold in the remaining sugar with a metal spoon. Pile on top of the lime pie and bake for 35 minutes until golden. Serve warm.

Treacle Tart

Corn flakes are an easy breadcrumb substitute and work very well in this traditional pudding. Outrageous with Praline Ice-cream (see page 180)!

Serves 6

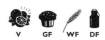

115g/4oz/³/₄ cup of rice flour
100g/3¹/₂ oz/²/₃ cup of maize flour
¹/₄ teaspoon of salt
140g/5oz/²/₃ cup of (DF) margarine
1 large egg yolk
3 heaped tablespoons of crushed 100% pure
   corn flakes

The grated rind of 1 lemon
The juice of ¹/₂ a lemon
7 rounded tablespoons of golden syrup (corn syrup)

23cm/9 inch fluted tart tin, greased and floured

Preheat the oven to 180°C/350°F/Gas mark 4

Sift the flours and salt into a mixing bowl. Cut the margarine into this using a blunt knife.
Mix in the egg yolk and a little cold water.
Bring together into a ball with floured fingers, then knead briefly on a floured board and roll out thickly.
Gently lift the pastry over the tart tin and press with your fingers to fit neatly. Trim the edges.
Sprinkle the corn flakes over the base and spoon over the lemon rind and juice.
Evenly distribute the syrup over it and bake in the oven for 25 minutes.
Let it get cold before serving warmed-up, otherwise it will be too crumbly. You can add chopped stem ginger for a change in the winter or serve with Stem Ginger Ice-cream (*see page 177*).

Plum Frangipani Tart

You can make this recipe with apricots in season, or even with greengages.

Serves 6

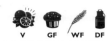

V GF WF DF

PASTRY

1 heaped tablespoon of icing (confectioners') sugar
Pinch of salt
70g/2¹/₂oz/¹/₂ cup of rice flour
70g/2¹/₂oz/¹/₂ cup of millet flour
70g/2¹/₂oz/¹/₂ cup of maize flour
140g/5oz/²/₃ cup of (DF) margarine
1 large free-range egg yolk

FRANGIPANE CREAM

70g/¹/₂oz/¹/₃ cup of caster (superfine) sugar
70g/2¹/₂oz/¹/₃ cup of (DF) margarine
55g/2oz/scant ¹/₂ cup of rice flour
2 large free-range eggs
150g/5oz/1²/₃ cups of ground almonds

1 tablespoon of orange flower water
¹/₂ teaspoon of almond essence

TOPPING

900g/32oz of fresh ripe plums, halved and stones (pits) removed

GLAZE

3 tablespoons of runny plum or apricot jam (jelly)
2 tablespoons of Amaretto di Saronno liqueur

25cm/10 inch loose-bottomed, fluted flan tin, greased and floured
Baking parchment (wax paper)
Ceramic baking beans

Preheat the oven to 190°C/375°F/Gas mark 5

First make the pastry. Mix all the ingredients briefly in a food processor until it comes together into a ball. Scrape out. Wrap in clingfilm (plastic wrap) and chill for 30 minutes. Then roll out the pastry to fit the flan tin. Cover with baking parchment (wax paper) and ceramic beans and bake blind for 20 minutes. Remove the beans and paper.

For the frangipane cream, mix all the ingredients briefly in a food processor until they are thick but not stiff. Add more orange water if necessary.

Cook the plums with a little water in a covered pan over a medium heat until a little softer and carefully drain off the juices.

Fill the cooked pastry shell with the frangipane cream and smooth over the top. Lay the plums, cut side down over the cream, starting around the edge and working into the middle. Bake for 40 minutes or until golden. Warm the jam (jelly) and Amaretto together and brush all over the tart. Serve warm.

Greengage and Almond Tart

This sweet, golden green fruit fuses all the late summer flavours together. Ambrosial when ripe, and a much neglected rival to the plum, they are worthy of the highest esteem from the severest critic.

Serves 10

PASTRY
115g/4oz/½ cup of (DF) margarine
55g/2oz/¼ cup of caster (superfine) sugar
1 large free-range egg, beaten
70g/2½oz/½ cup of rice flour
70g/2½oz/½ cup of maize flour
½ teaspoon of ground cinnamon
½ teaspoon of ground allspice
A pinch of salt
1 heaped tablespoon of millet flakes

ALMOND CREAM
85g/3oz/6 tablespoons of (DF) margarine
85g/3oz/6 tablespoons of caster (superfine) sugar

2 large free-range eggs
1 tablespoon of dark rum
85g/3oz/1 cup of ground almonds
20g/¾oz/2 generous tablespoons of rice flour

FRUIT FILLING
680g/1½lb of fresh and very ripe greengages, stalks
  removed
4 tablespoons of apricot jam (jelly) warmed in a pan
  with 1 tablespoon of dark rum

32cm/12½inch loose-bottomed, fluted tart tin,
  greased and floured

Preheat the oven to 200°C/400°F/Gas mark 6

First make the pastry. Beat the margarine and the sugar together in a food processor and add enough egg to make a wet paste. Sift the flours, spices and salt into the dough, add the millet flakes and process briefly in order to blend together. When the dough comes together into a ball, wrap it in clingfilm (plastic wrap) and chill for 30 minutes in the deep freeze.
Roll out the pastry on a floured board and carefully line the tin with it, pushing the pastry into shape with floured fingers. Trim the edges with a knife and discard the remnants.
Beat the margarine and sugar until pale and fluffy, then mix in the eggs and rum. Fold in the almonds, sieve in the flour and mix gently. Cover the base of the tart with the mixture.
Halve the greengages, stone (pit) them and arrange them close together over the almond cream. Bake the tart for 45 minutes, or until the fruit is puffy and golden. The fruit should be just soft but not bursting. Remove the tart from the oven and leave it in the tin to cool.
Dissolve the jam and rum together in a bowl in the microwave and spread it over the fruit tart. Leave the tart to cool before removing it from the tin onto a plate. Serve the tart just warm. You can reheat the tart if you are making it in advance, but it should be served fresh and warm.

Pear Tart Tatin

French chefs use pears or apples for this lovely pudding. It is heavenly served with home-made (DF)
vanilla ice-cream.

Serves 6

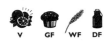

PASTRY
100g/3¹/₂oz/²/₃ cup of rice flour
70g/2¹/₂oz/¹/₂ cup of maize flour
55g/2oz/¹/₃ cup of ground rice
140g/5oz/²/₃ cup of (DF) margarine
55g/2oz/scant ¹/₄ cup of caster (superfine) sugar
1 large free-range egg, beaten

TOPPING
100g/3¹/₂oz/¹/₂ cup of (DF) margarine
140g/5oz/7 tablespoons of granulated sugar
1.05kg/37oz/7¹/₂ cups of ripe pears, peeled, cored
   and quartered
The grated rind of 1 lemon

Tart Tatin dish or a 25cm/10 inch deep, round
   baking tin

Preheat the oven to 200°C/400°F/Gas mark 6

First make the pastry. Sift the flours and ground rice together into a large bowl, then rub in the
margarine until it resembles fine breadcrumbs. Stir in the sugar and add the egg. Mix until you
have a binding dough. Wrap in clingfilm (plastic wrap) and chill until needed.
Now make the topping. Gently melt the margarine in a large frying pan (skillet) with the sugar.
Turn up the heat to high and once the margarine and sugar have started to boil add the pears to
the pan. Sprinkle the lemon rind over the pears.
Cook until the margarine starts to caramelize. Remove from the heat.
Put all the pears with the caramel into the dish. Roll out the pastry on a floured board into a thick
circle, to fit the top of the pan. Lay it on top of the pears and press down slightly.
Bake in the oven for 10 minutes and then reduce the oven temperature to 190°C/375°F/Gas mark
5 and bake for a further 10 minutes, until golden and bubbling.
Allow to cool slightly before turning onto a warm plate and serving.

Plum Tatin

Luckily, this recipe exploits the virtues of unripe plums. As supermarkets seldom seem to sell fruit that is ripe enough, it is the perfect solution.

Serves 6

PASTRY
100g/3¹/₂oz/²/₃ cup of rice flour
70g/2¹/₂oz/¹/₂ cup of maize flour
55g/2oz/¹/₃ cup of ground rice
140g/5oz/²/₃ cup (DF) margarine
55g/2oz/¹/₄ cup of caster (superfine) sugar
1 free-range egg, beaten

TOPPING
130g/4¹/₂oz/¹/₂ cup plus 1 tablespoon of (DF) margarine
130g/4¹/₂oz/generous ¹/₂ cup of caster (superfine) sugar mixed with 1 tablespoon of ground cinnamon
1kg/2lb 2oz of Victoria plums, wiped clean

Tart Tatin mould or a 25cm/10 inch non-stick, round baking tin

Preheat the oven to 200°C/400°F/Gas mark 6

First make the pastry. Sift the flours and the ground rice together into a large bowl and rub in the margarine until the mixture resembles fine breadcrumbs. Stir in the sugar, add the egg and mix until you have a binding dough. Wrap in clingfilm (plastic wrap) and chill until needed.
Melt the margarine for the topping in a large frying pan (skillet) with the sugar and cinnamon. Halve the plums and remove the stones (pits). Place the plums in the frying pan (skillet) and increase the heat to high.
Cook the plums until the margarine and sugar starts to caramelize. Quickly remove the pan from the heat and transfer the fruit and juices to the tatin dish.
Roll out the pastry on a floured surface into a thick circle large enough to fit over the plums. Lay the pastry over the fruit and press down slightly.
Bake in the oven for 25–30 minutes, or until the pastry is golden and the fruit cooked and bubbling. Serve warm with (DF) vanilla ice-cream.

Rhubarb and Pistachio Crumble

Pistachios are such fun to nibble at when they are fresh in their shells and easy to crack open and pop into one's mouth. A packet of shelled nuts will do perfectly well for this recipe and the pistachios will add a touch of sophistication to the crumble.

Serves 8

600g/1lb 3oz/4½ cups of fresh trimmed rhubarb, washed and chopped

4 tablespoons of sugar

¾ teaspoon of ground cinnamon

2 whole cloves

2 tablespoons of ginger wine or ginger cordial

100g/3½ oz/7 tablespoons of (DF) margarine

85g/3oz/9 tablespoons of rice flour

85g/3oz/1 cup of millet flakes

4 tablespoons of demerara sugar

100g/3½ oz/¾ cup of shelled pistachio nuts, roughly chopped

Sugar for sprinkling

Preheat the oven to 190°C/375°F/Gas mark 5

Put the rhubarb, sugar, cinnamon, cloves and ginger wine or cordial into a deep pan and cook gently until just soft. Stir occasionally to prevent sticking.

Make the crumble in a bowl by rubbing the margarine into the flour and millet flakes with your fingertips. Stir in the demerara sugar and nuts.

Remove the cloves from the rhubarb and discard.

Spoon the fruit into an ovenproof pie dish, leaving behind the excess juices. Pour the crumble over the fruit and sprinkle the top with the sugar.

Bake for 40 minutes, or until the crumble is crispy and the rhubarb is bubbling up. Serve hot with Zabaglione (*see page 119*) or some (DF) vanilla ice-cream.

Apple and Blackberry Crumble

This good old-fashioned pudding is delicious served with Coconut Ice-cream (see page 178) or Ginger Custard (see page 133).

Serves 6

V / WF DF

4 large cooking apples
4 tablespoons of sugar
1 teaspoon of (GF) mixed (pie) spice
The juice of ¹/₂ a lemon
500g/17oz/3¹/₂ cups of fresh or frozen blackberries
1 teaspoon of (DF) margarine

CRUMBLE
115g/4oz/¹/₂ cup of (DF) margarine
55g/2oz/¹/₃ cup of sugar
55g/2oz/¹/₂ cup of oats
100g/3¹/₂oz/²/₃ cup of rice flour
55g/2oz/¹/₂ cup of millet flakes
1 teaspoon of ground cinnamon

Deep-sided 30cm/12 inch ovenproof dish

Preheat the oven to 180°C/350°F/Gas mark 4

Peel and core the apples and slice finely. Place in a saucepan with the sugar, mixed (pie) spice and lemon juice and cook gently until soft. Add the blackberries and remove from the heat. Dot with margarine.

Next make the crumble using the food processor by mixing the margarine with the sugar for a few seconds. Add the oats, rice, flour, millet flakes and cinnamon and whiz briefly together.

Put the apple mixture into the ovenproof dish, cover with the crumble and bake in the centre of the oven for 25 minutes, or until golden and bubbling.

Hot Pear Brownie

Chocolate and pears are always a good combination, hot or cold. This is a slightly healthier version of other sticky puddings.

Serves 6

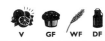

820g/30oz/4 cups of pears in fruit juice
70g/2½oz/½ cup of rice flour
A pinch of salt
1 teaspoon of (GF) baking powder
70g/2½oz/⅓ cup of (DF) margarine

½ teaspoon of vanilla essence
70g/2½oz of (DF/GF) dark chocolate
170g/6oz/generous ¾ cup of caster (superfine) sugar
2 large free-range eggs, beaten
70g/2½oz/⅔ cup of chopped pecan nuts

Preheat the oven to 180°C/350°F/Gas mark 4

Grease a deep baking dish. Cover the base with the pears.
Sift the flour, salt and baking powder into a bowl. Put the margarine, vanilla essence and chocolate into a saucepan, stir until melted and then remove from the heat.
Beat in the sugar, eggs and pecans. Stir the chocolate mixture into the dry ingredients, pour the batter over the pears and bake in the centre of the oven for about 35 minutes or until the brownie mix is just firm.
Serve warm with (DF) ice-cream or Zabaglione (*see page 119*) for a dinner party.

Rum and Chocolate Bread Pudding

This captures the essence of traditional British food but is transformed into a contemporary dish with the addition of rum and chocolate. Any leftovers can be eaten cold the next day with (DF) vanilla ice-cream.

Serves 6

V GF WF DF

170g/6oz (about 6 slices) of (GF) white bread, (available from health food stores and by mail order)
240ml/8fl oz/1 cup of soya cream
100ml/3½ fl oz/⅓ cup of soya milk
140g/5oz of (DF/GF) continental dark chocolate
55g/2oz/scant ¼ cup of caster sugar
55g/2oz/¼ cup of (DF) margarine

1 teaspoon of ground cinnamon
5 tablespoons of dark rum
3 large free-range eggs
1 teaspoon of pure Madagascan vanilla extract

26 x 19 x 5cm/10½ x 7½ x 2 inch ovenproof dish, oiled

Preheat the oven to 180°C/350°F/Gas mark 4

Remove the crusts from the bread and cut the bread squares into triangles. Put the soya cream and milk, chocolate, sugar, margarine and cinnamon into a bowl. Place the bowl over a pan of simmering water until the sugar has dissolved and the mixture melted. Stir in the rum.
In a separate bowl, whisk the eggs and pour them into the chocolate mixture. Add the vanilla extract and whisk the eggs again.
Spoon one third of the mixture into the dish and arrange the bread triangles over it, overlapping and pointed side up. Pour in the remainder of the chocolate mixture and, using a wooden spoon, gently press down the bread to ensure that all the bread is submerged.
Leave to stand for 2 hours and then transfer it to the refrigerator for 4 hours. Keep the bowl covered with clingfilm (plastic wrap).
Pour some water into a shallow baking tin and stand the bread and butter pudding dish in it. Bake for 40–45 minutes until puffed up in the centre. Allow to stand for 10 minutes before eating.

Pear and Blackberry Eve's Pudding

I am so glad that blackberries are being cultivated for supermarkets now, as they are fiendishly difficult to pick amidst all the prickly brambles that grow in the ditches and along windy country lanes. Alas, they are usually covered in exhaust fumes as well!

Serves 8

V   WF   DF

---

2 × 425g/15oz cans of pears in natural juice
340g/12oz/2½ cups of fresh or frozen blackberries
½ teaspoon of (GF) mixed (pie) spice
140g/5oz/⅔ cup of (DF) margarine
140g/5oz/¾ cup of light brown sugar
70g/2½oz/½ cup of barley flour

70g/2½oz/½ cup of rice flour
55g/2oz/⅔ cup of ground almonds
2 large free-range eggs, beaten
2 tablespoons of the drained pear juice
2 teaspoons of (GF) baking powder
2 tablespoons of pine nuts

Preheat the oven to 190°C/375°F/Gas mark 5

Drain the pears, reserving two tablespoons of the juice for the pudding. Slice the pears and arrange them in a large ovenproof baking dish. Cover with the blackberries and sprinkle with the mixed (pie) spice.

In a food processor, beat the margarine with the brown sugar until light and fluffy. Add the flours and ground almonds and briefly combine. Mix the eggs and pear juice together in a small bowl and then blend them briefly into the flour mixture. Finally, fold in the baking powder and gently spread the mixture over the fruit.

Sprinkle the pudding with the pine nuts and bake in the oven for about 40–50 minutes, or until the sponge is browned and just firm to touch.

Serve the pudding hot with (DF) ice-cream or Zabaglione (*see page 119*).

Blackcurrant Rice Surprise

Nursery puddings, although we hate to admit it, are so very reassuring! Now that trendy restaurants are serving old-fashioned puddings once again, we can all enjoy them.

Serves 6

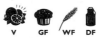

30g/1oz/2 tablespoons of (DF) margarine

300ml/10fl oz/1¼ cups of coconut milk

300ml/10fl oz/1¼ cups of soya milk

300ml/10fl oz/1¼ cups of water

100g/3½oz/½ cup of pudding rice

30g/1oz/2 tablespoons of caster (superfine) sugar

255g/9oz/1¾ cups of fresh or frozen trimmed blackcurrants

3 tablespoons of caster (superfine) sugar

3 large free-range eggs, separated

1 teaspoon of pure Madagascan vanilla extract

100g/3½oz/½ cup of caster (superfine) sugar

Preheat the oven to 180°C/350°F/Gas mark 4

Melt the margarine with the coconut milk and soya milk in a non-stick saucepan over low heat. Add the water, rice and 30g/1oz/2 tablespoons of caster (superfine) sugar, and increase the heat to medium. Bring the pan of rice to the boil, stirring occasionally, then simmer over low heat for about 45 minutes until just soft, thick and creamy.

Meanwhile, mix the fruit and 3 tablespoons of sugar together.

Once the rice is done, remove from the heat and stir in the egg yolks and vanilla extract. Spoon the rice into a deep-sided, ovenproof dish big enough for six servings and level it off. Spoon all the sweetened blackcurrants over the rice.

Make the meringue topping. Whisk the egg whites in a large bowl until stiff, then fold in the 100g/3½oz/½ cup of caster (superfine) sugar. Spread gently over the blackcurrants and bake for about 30 minutes, or until well browned.

Serve the pudding either hot or warm.

Blueberry Sponge Pudding with Zabaglione

Steamed sponge puddings have been back in vogue for a few years now. This very traditional English family pudding is economical and easy to make – perfect for the harassed parent battling his or her way through the preparations for Sunday lunch. Here the pudding is served with Zabaglione, but for an even simpler accompaniment try golden syrup (corn syrup).

Serves 8

V   GF   WF   DF

4 heaped tablespoons of blueberry jam (jelly)

255g/9oz/1³/4 cups of fresh blueberries, washed and dried

100g/3¹/2oz/7 tablespoons of (DF) margarine

100g/3¹/2oz/¹/2 cup of caster (superfine) sugar

2 large free-range eggs, beaten

1 teaspoon of pure Madagascan vanilla extract

100g/3¹/2oz/²/3 cup of rice flour

100g/3¹/2oz/²/3 cup of maize flour

2 teaspoons of (GF) baking powder

Apple juice to mix

Greased baking parchment (wax paper) and some string

900ml/1¹/2 pints/3³/4 cup pudding basin, greased with (DF) margarine and dusted with (GF) flour

ZABAGLIONE

4 large free-range egg yolks

70g/2¹/2 oz/¹/3 cup of caster (superfine) sugar

100ml/3¹/2 fl oz/¹/3 cup of Marsala

First make the pudding. Half fill a large saucepan with water and put it on to boil. Spoon half the jam (jelly) into the bottom of the prepared pudding basin, cover with half of the blueberries and then spoon on the remaining jam (jelly).

Cream together the margarine and sugar in a food processor for 1 minute. Add the eggs and vanilla and process briefly. Briefly blend in the flours and baking powder. Add the apple juice to soften it to a dropping consistency and fold in the remaining blueberries. Scrape the mixture immediately into the pudding basin. Cover with greased baking parchment (wax paper), making a central pleat in the paper to allow the pudding to expand. Secure the paper by tying string firmly around the rim of the bowl, making a little handle so you can lift the pudding out of the water more easily. Steam, with the saucepan tightly covered, for 1¹/2 hours (topping up the water level when necessary). Carefully lift the pudding our of the saucepan and leave it to settle while you make the Zabaglione.

Fill another saucepan one third of the way up with water and bring it to the boil. Put the egg yolks and sugar into a large heatproof bowl and beat together with an electric whisk. Now add the Marsala. Put the bowl over the saucepan of simmering water and whisk on high speed until very thick. Serve immediately. Turn the blueberry pudding out onto a large serving plate and serve immediately with the warm sauce.

Apple and Cranberry Streusel Pudding

The combinations of fruits used in restaurants can be illuminating but also sometimes a little too precious! This is a traditional and festive mixture of fruits, perfect for our bleak mid-winter. Use ripe pears instead of the apples for a change.

Serves 6

140g/5oz/²/₃ cup of (DF) margarine

140g/5oz/³/₄ cup of caster (superfine) sugar

2 large free-range eggs, beaten

Finely grated zest and juice of 1 lemon

70g/2¹/₂oz/¹/₂ cup of barley flour

55g/2oz/scant ¹/₂ cup of oat flour (finely process flaked oats if necessary)

2 teaspoons of (GF) baking powder

45g/1¹/₂oz/¹/₂ cup of ground almonds

TOPPING

3 large dessert apples, peeled, quartered, cored and sliced

255g/9oz/2¹/₄ cups of fresh or frozen cranberries

115g/4oz/¹/₂ cup of soft brown sugar

70g/2¹/₂oz/¹/₂ cup of oat flour

55g/2oz/²/₃ cup of ground almonds

55g/2oz/¹/₄ cup of sunflower margarine

Finely grated zest of 1 lemon

1 heaped teaspoon of ground cinnamon

¹/₂ teaspoon of grated nutmeg

¹/₂ teaspoon of ground cardamom

23cm/9 inch loose-bottomed cake tin, greased with some (DF) margarine

Preheat the oven to 190°C/375°F/Gas mark 5

Cream the margarine and sugar in a food processor and gradually beat in the eggs. Transfer to a bowl, mix in the lemon zest and fold in the flours and baking powder. Gently stir in the ground almonds and lemon juice and then spread the mixture lightly over the bottom of the cake tin. To make the topping, toss the apples and cranberries with 70g/2¹/₂oz/5 tablespoons of the soft brown sugar in a bowl. Spread the fruit over the cake base. Put the remaining soft brown sugar, flour and ground almonds into a bowl and rub in the margarine. Mix in the lemon zest and spices, and spread the mixture over the fruit.
Bake for about 1¹/₂ hours, or until the apples are soft and the streusel browned and crunchy.

Baked Ginger Pudding and Marsala Ice-cream

This reminds me of the school holidays when we used to have something very like this as a treat, but unfortunately not with the addition of Marsala!

Serves 6

V · GF · WF · DF

ICE-CREAM
4 large free-range egg yolks
1 teaspoon of (GF) cornflour (cornstarch)
85g/3oz/6 tablespoons of caster (superfine) sugar
1/4 teaspoon of ground cinnamon
500ml/17fl oz/2 cups of soya cream
90ml/3fl oz/1/3 cup of Marsala

PUDDING
100g/3 1/2 oz/2/3 cup of rice flour
2 teaspoons of ground cinnamon
1 teaspoon of ground ginger
A pinch of ground cloves
Freshly grated nutmeg
1 teaspoon of bicarbonate of soda (baking soda)

100g/3 1/2 oz/1/2 cup of soft dark brown sugar
1 large free-range egg
140ml/5fl oz/2/3 cup of Marsala
75g/3oz/1/4 cup of black treacle (molasses)
55g/2oz/1/4 cup of (DF) margarine, melted
Zest of 1 large orange
100g/3 1/2 oz/3/4 cup of stem ginger, drained and chopped or sugar-coated ginger pieces
85g/3oz/1/2 cup of plump raisins
Extra grated nutmeg and ground cinnamon for decoration

A large, terrine tin or loaf tin, lined with baking parchment (wax paper)

Preheat the oven to 180°C/350°F/Gas mark 4

Make the ice-cream first. Whisk the egg yolks with the cornflour (cornstarch) and caster sugar. Add the cinnamon and cream and cook in a non-stick saucepan over low heat until it reaches boiling point. Do not let it boil. Remove the pan from the heat and quickly stir in the Marsala. Allow the mixture to cool, stirring it occasionally to prevent a skin forming.

Transfer the mixture to the ice-cream maker and churn until frozen. This will probably take about 20 minutes.

Scrape the ice-cream into a sealable container and freeze for 2–4 hours before serving with the pudding.

Make the pudding. Sieve the flour into a bowl along with the spices, bicarbonate of soda (baking soda) and sugar. Beat in the egg, followed by the Marsala, treacle (molasses), melted margarine and orange zest. Stir in the ginger and raisins.

Pour the mixture into the prepared tin and bake for 35 minutes. Have the ice-cream at room temperature 10 minutes before serving.

Turn the cake out of the tin and peel off the baking parchment (wax paper). Cut the cake into thick slices, place a slice on each plate with a scoop of ice-cream and sprinkle with a little grated nutmeg and ground cinnamon.

Chocolate Topsy Turvy Pudding

This wonderful concoction is a scientific mystery, the chocolate sauce on top of the cake magically sinks down and appears as a sauce at the bottom of the cake. My God-children love it!

Serves 6

V   GF WF DF

100g/3½oz/⅔ cup of rice flour
1 heaped teaspoon of (GF) baking powder
5 tablespoons of (DF/GF) cocoa powder
A pinch of salt
55g/2oz/½ cup of chopped walnuts
115g/4oz/½ cup of (DF) margarine
115g/4oz/½ cup plus 1 tablespoon of caster (superfine) sugar
2 large free-range eggs

1 teaspoon of pure Madagascan vanilla extract
115g/4oz/½ cup plus 1 tablespoon of soft brown sugar
4 tablespoons of rum
240ml/8fl oz/1 cup of boiling water

1½ litre/2 pint/3 US pint soufflé dish, greased with (DF) margarine and dusted with a little caster (superfine) sugar

Preheat the oven to 190°C/375°F/Gas mark 5

Sift the flour, baking powder, 1 tablespoon of the cocoa powder and the salt into a bowl, then fold in the walnuts.

In another large bowl, beat the margarine and sugar until pale and light, add the eggs and vanilla extract and then mix in the sifted dry ingredients.

Spoon the mixture into the prepared soufflé dish and level off.

Mix the brown sugar with the remaining cocoa and the rum, and dissolve them with the boiling water. Pour the sauce over the cake and then bake for 30–35 minutes, or until the sponge is just firm and the sauce has sunk to the bottom.

Serve warm on its own or with (DF) vanilla ice-cream.

Nectarine and Apricot Clafoutis

You can vary the fruit in this recipe throughout the year, using fresh or canned and drained, apricots, cherries, blackberries or prunes. Serve warm rather than hot.

Serves 8

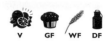

3 ripe nectarines, peeled, stoned (pitted) and cut into sixths
Juice of ½ a lemon
Icing (confectioners') sugar to dust

BATTER
20g/¾oz/3 tablespoons of rice flour
A pinch of salt
115g/4oz/½ cup plus 1 tablespoon of caster (superfine) sugar

60ml/2fl oz/¼ cup of Amaretto liqueur
Grated rind of 1 lemon
4 large free-range eggs
240ml/8fl oz/1 cup of soya cream

A deep-sided 28 x 20cm/11 x 8 inch ovenproof china dish, generously greased with (DF) margarine and dusted with rice flour

Preheat the oven to 190°C/375°F/Gas mark 5

Put the nectarines and the lemon juice in a bowl together. Make the batter by blending the flour, salt, sugar, liqueur and lemon rind together in a bowl. Gradually incorporate the eggs, followed by the cream.
Shake the excess flour off the prepared dish and arrange the nectarines over the base of the dish.
Mix the remaining lemon juice into the batter and then pour it over the fruit.
Bake in the oven for 40 minutes, or until firm and golden.
Dust the Clafoutis with icing (confectioners') sugar to serve.

Little Toffee Apple Puddings

Give in to temptation and enjoy the glories of English apples baked with a hint of spices and lemon rind. I do not use cooking apples because they are too tart, so treat yourself to an old fashioned eating apple instead.

Serves 6

APPLES IN CARAMEL

2 medium dessert apples, peeled, quartered, cored, finely sliced horizontally and soaked in the juice of 1 lemon

115g/4oz/½ cup plus 1 tablespoon of caster (superfine) sugar

200ml/7fl oz/¾ cup of water

60ml/2fl oz/¼ cup of dry cider

55g/2oz/¼ cup of dark muscovado sugar

30g/1oz/2 tablespoons of (DF) margarine

SPONGE

A pinch of salt

130g/4½oz/generous ¾ cup of rice flour

130g/4½oz/generous ¾ cup of maize flour

2 teaspoons of (GF) baking powder

55g/2oz/4 tablespoons of light brown sugar

1 teaspoon of ground cinnamon

1 teaspoon of ground ginger

½ teaspoon of ground cloves

½ teaspoon of allspice

2 tablespoons of runny honey

1 large free-range egg

140ml/5fl oz/⅔ cup of dry cider

125ml/4fl oz/½ cup of vegetable or sunflower oil

Grated zest of 1 lemon

6 ovenproof ramekins, lightly oiled and placed on a baking tray

---

Preheat the oven to 180°C/350°F/Gas mark 4

Make sure you have the apples and lemon juice ready for the recipe.

Place the caster (superfine) sugar and water in a saucepan over medium heat and stir gently until the sugar has dissolved. Increase the heat to high and bring to the boil. Let the sugar syrup caramelize into pale golden brown colour but remove the caramel from the heat as soon as it starts to get dark or it will taste bitter. Immediately pour in the cider and beware of spluttering caramel. Set aside while you cook the apples.

Heat the muscovado sugar and margarine in a saucepan until they melt and dissolve together. Add the apples and cook over medium heat until the apples are nearly soft and coated with the sauce. As soon as most of the sauce has evaporated, stir in all the cider caramel.

Divide the mixture between the 6 prepared ramekins, then set them aside while you prepare the sponge.

Sift the dry ingredients and spices into a large bowl. In another bowl, mix the honey, egg, cider, oil and lemon zest. Stir the wet mixture into the dry mixture and immediately spoon it onto the caramelized apples in each ramekin. Gently smooth over the top and bake in the oven for 25–30 minutes, or until the sponge is golden and firm.

Let the sponges cool just enough for you to be able to hold the ramekins in a dry cloth. Ease the sponge away from the sides of the dish with a sharp knife, then turn each one onto a warm plate and serve immediately with (DF) vanilla ice-cream or (DF) yogurt.

Pineapple Cake

Thai food has brought lemon grass to our attention and now we cannot get enough of it. Use canned pineapple if you are short of time, but make sure it is in natural fruit juices, otherwise the pudding becomes too sweet and bland. If you prefer a richer taste, use dark rum in place of the white.

Serves 8

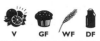

CAKE

170g/6oz/³/4 cup of (DF) margarine, plus extra for greasing

170g/6oz/³/4 cup of caster (superfine) sugar

Finely grated rind of 1 lemon

3 large free-range eggs, separated

85g/3oz/9 tablespoons of rice flour

75ml/2¹/2fl oz/¹/4 cup total combined mixture of the above lemon, juiced and some white rum

85g/3oz/1 cup of ground almonds

1 teaspoon of (GF) baking powder

SYRUP AND DECORATION

2 sticks of fresh lemon grass, trimmed of tough outer layer and ends

30g/1oz/2 tablespoons of granulated sugar

Juice of 1 lemon

3 tablespoons of white rum

1 large ripe pineapple, peeled and trimmed, cut into quarters, cored and chopped into slices

Sunflower oil for frying the pineapple

22cm/8³/4 inch non-stick ring mould cake tin, greased

Preheat the oven to 170°C/325°F/Gas mark 3

Beat the margarine and caster sugar in a food processor until pale and fluffy. Add the finely grated lemon rind to the mixture. Gradually beat in the egg yolks, followed by 2 tablespoons of the flour and the lemon juice and rum mixture. Transfer the mixture to a large bowl and lightly fold in half of the almonds and half the remaining flour.

Now fold in the remaining almonds, the last of the flour and the baking powder. Whisk the egg whites until they form firm peaks. Quickly fold the egg whites into the prepared mixture.

Spoon the mixture into the tin and bake in the oven for about 50 minutes, or until an inserted skewer comes out clean.

Allow the cake to cool slightly, then turn it out onto a wire rack to cool completely.

While the cake is baking, slice the lemon grass very finely and place in a pan with the 30g/1oz/2 tablespoons of sugar and 200ml/7fl oz/³/4 cup of water. Simmer for 10 minutes over low heat. Increase the heat to high, bring the syrup to the boil for 2–3 minutes and then add the lemon juice and the rum. Strain the syrup and discard the lemon grass.

Place the cake on a serving plate, prick small holes all over the cake and pour the syrup all over it. Just before serving, fry the pineapple slices in the sunflower oil. (If you use a char-grill pan the slices will have trendy grill marks on them). They should be just softened with a few char marks. Pile the hot pineapple into the central hole of the cake and serve immediately.

Warm Butterscotch Pear Cake

Serve this cake warm with (DF) vanilla ice-cream or your choice of (DF) natural or vanilla yogurt. You can also successfully make this recipe with sweet dessert apples.

Serves 12

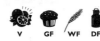

CAKE

2 large, just-ripe pears, peeled, quartered, cored and
   thinly sliced into the juice of 1 lemon
200g/7oz/1 cup less 2 tablespoons of (DF) margarine
170g/6oz/generous ¾ cup of caster (superfine) sugar
2 large free-range eggs
130g/4½oz/generous ¾ cup of rice flour
100g/3½oz/⅔ cup of maize flour
A pinch of salt
3 teaspoons of (GF) baking powder
1 heaped teaspoon of ground ginger
1 teaspoon of freshly grated nutmeg
140ml/5fl oz/⅔ cup of dry ginger ale
Finely grated zest of 1 lemon
55g/2oz/⅔ cup of ground almonds

TOPPING

55g/2oz/¼ cup of (DF) margarine
115g/4oz/½ cup plus 1 tablespoon of muscovado
   sugar
Few drops of pure Madagascan vanilla extract
100g/3½oz/1 cup of flaked almonds
Icing (confectioners') sugar to dust

25cm/10 inch loose-bottomed, spring-form,
   round cake tin, greased and lined with baking
   parchment (wax paper)

Preheat the oven to 180°C/350°F/Gas mark 4

Ensure the pears are prepared before beginning the cake. In a food processor, cream together the margarine and caster (superfine) sugar until pale and fluffy, then beat in the eggs. Sift together the flours with the salt, baking powder, ginger and nutmeg and briefly blend into the egg mixture. Quickly add the ginger ale, lemon zest and ground almonds, and process for a moment only.
Remove the blade of the food processor and fold in half the pears in the juice.
Spoon half the cake mixture into the prepared tin and gently smooth over.
Cover the sponge with all the remaining pears and juice. Cover the pears with the remaining sponge mixture and smooth over.
Bake the cake for 40 minutes, or until golden and fairly firm.
Meanwhile, put the margarine and sugar together into a pan over medium heat and cook gently until the sugar dissolves, about 3–4 minutes will be enough. Bring it to the boil and then add the vanilla extract and flaked almonds. Remove from the heat and stir the mixture.
Take the cake out of the oven and spread the almond mixture over the top of the cake.
Return the cake to the oven for about 15–20 minutes, or until the topping is sticky and the sponge is firm.

Leave the cake in the tin to cool for at least 40 minutes, then carefully remove the cake from the tin and peel off the lining paper.

Place the cake on a plate and dust with sieved icing (confectioners') sugar. Serve it just warm with ice-cream or yogurt.

Festive Apple and Mincemeat Meringue

This is an excellent alternative to slaving over heaps of mince pies at Christmas and avoids the hassle of making lots of pastry.

Serves 8

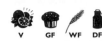

1kg/2.2lb of large cooking apples, washed and dried

1 heaped teaspoon of ground cinnamon

Grated zest of 1 lemon

55g/2oz/4 tablespoons of dark brown sugar

2 tablespoons of Calvados or brandy

825g/1lb 13oz/2½ cups of deluxe (GF/DF) vegetarian mincemeat

4 large free-range egg whites

A pinch of salt

200g/7oz/1 cup of caster (superfine) sugar

55g/2oz/²/₃ cup of ground almonds

55g/2oz/²/₃ cup of flaked almonds

Ground cinnamon and icing (confectioners') sugar sifted together to dust

Preheat the oven to 150°C/300°F/Gas mark 2

Peel and core the apples, chop up into little cubes and place in a saucepan with the cinnamon, lemon zest, brown sugar and Calvados. Cook for 5 minutes over medium heat, stirring frequently so that the apples do not stick to the pan.

Transfer the mixture to a deep ovenproof dish and level off the top. Spread the mincemeat evenly over the apples.

In a large bowl, whisk the egg whites and salt at high speed until stiff peaks form. Reduce the speed to low and whisk in the 200g/7oz/1 cup of sugar. When the meringue is firm and glossy, gently fold in the ground almonds. Pile the meringue over the mincemeat.

Sprinkle with the flaked almonds and bake for 30–40 minutes until golden and crisp.

Serve dusted with cinnamon and icing (confectioners') sugar.

Christmas Pudding

This pudding can be made up to one week in advance, which is so useful during the chaotic run-up to Christmas day.

Makes 1 very large, or 2 medium puddings

70g/2¹/²oz/¹/³ cup of glacé cherries, chopped
170g/6oz/1 cup of candied peel, chopped
340g/12oz/2¹/² cups of raisins
170g/6oz/1¹/⁴ cups of sultanas (golden raisins)
170g/6oz/1¹/⁴ cups of currants
70g/2¹/²oz/¹/² cup of blanched almonds, chopped
255g/9oz/2 cups of 100% (GF) corn breadcrumbs or (WF) rye breadcrumbs
255g/9oz/2 cups of (GF) shredded vegetarian suet
2 heaped teaspoons of ground cinnamon
2 heaped teaspoons (GF) mixed (pie) spice
¹/² of a nutmeg, grated

¹/² teaspoon of ground cloves
1 teaspoon of allspice
6 large free-range eggs
Grated rind and juice of 1 orange
Grated rind of ¹/² a lemon
140ml/5fl oz/²/³ cup of Armagnac or brandy
3 tablespoons of rum
Sunflower oil for greasing

2 litre/3¹/⁴ pint/2 quart pudding basin or 2 × 1 litre/1³/⁴ pint/1 quart basins, generously oiled
Baking foil and string

Put the dried fruit, almonds, breadcrumbs, suet and spices into a large bowl and mix together. Whisk the eggs until fluffy and thickened, then stir into the dry ingredients. Blend in the grated orange and its juice, the grated lemon and spirits. The mixture should just drop off the spoon. Put the mixture into the pudding basin(s) and smooth over the top. Cover the basin with a layer of oiled foil, double folded in the centre, and secure with string.

Stand the basin on an inverted saucer or a piece of foil folded 4 times, in a very large saucepan. Fill three quarters of the way up with water, cover with a lid or foil and steam for 6¹/² hours for a large pudding or 4¹/² hours for a smaller one. Top up with boiling water whenever necessary. When cooked, lift the basin out of the pan and allow to cool. Store in a cool dark place.

To reheat, replace the old foil with new foil and steam for 1¹/²–2 hours before serving.

Serve with Zabaglione (*see page 119*) or Ginger Custard (*see page 133*).

Mince Pies and Ginger Custard

Commercial mincemeat is often too sweet and has a less distinctive texture than the home-made variety. This version is fresh and fruity and can be made anytime from a couple of months before Christmas, to the day before.

Makes 48 pies

  or

V   GF   WF DF

PASTRY

310g/11oz/scant 2¼ cups of (GF) maize flour or millet flour

310g/11oz/scant 2¼ cups of rice flour

310g/11oz/scant 2¼ cups of finely processed (WF) oats, or (GF) maize or millet flour (use the opposite of the first ingredient choice)

480g/17oz/2¼ cups of (DF) margarine

½ teaspoon of salt

2 large free-range eggs, beaten

Some water to bind the dough

FINISHING TOUCHES

Caster (superfine) sugar and ground cinnamon for dusting

Icing (confectioners') sugar

MINCEMEAT

1.5kg/3.3lb/4½ cups of commercial vegetarian (GF/DF) mincemeat

or

170g/6oz/1¼ cups of currants

170g/6oz/1¼ cups of raisins, chopped finely

170g/6oz/1¼ cups of sultanas (golden raisins), chopped finely

115g/4oz/⅔ cup of prunes, chopped finely

170g/6oz/1 cup of dried apples, chopped finely

115g/4oz/⅔ cup of glacé cherries, chopped finely

115g/4oz/⅔ cup of candied peel, chopped finely

250g/8½oz/2 cups of (GF) vegetarian suet

300g/10½oz/1½ cups of light brown muscovado sugar

1 teaspoon of ground cloves

2 teaspoons of (GF) mixed (pie) spice

Grated rind and juice of 2 lemons

240ml/8fl oz/1 cup of Grand Marnier

Grated rind of 1 orange

1 ripe pear, peeled, cored and chopped

115g/4oz/⅔ cup of fresh cranberries, chopped

GINGER CUSTARD

For 6–8 people (double the quantities for 12–16 people)

6 large free-range egg yolks

100g/3½oz/½ cup of caster (superfine) sugar

1 tablespoon of (GF) cornflour (cornstarch)

3 tablespoons of stem ginger syrup

600ml/20fl oz/2½ cups of unsweetened soya milk

3 tablespoons of Stones' ginger wine, or rum

4 x 12-hole patty tins, greased, floured and lined with circles of baking parchment (wax paper)

Preheat the oven to 180°C/350°F/Gas mark 4

To make the mincemeat, put all of the dried fruit, cherries and candied peel into a large mixing bowl. Add the suet, sugar, spices, lemon rind and juice, grated orange rind and Grand Marnier.

Stir in the mincemeat thoroughly and add more liqueur if not moist.

Spoon the mixture into sterilised jars, cover and leave in a cold place for 2 days or use now to make the mince pies by mixing in the chopped pear and chopped cranberries.

To make the pastry, mix all of the ingredients, except the water, in the food processor, blending for a few seconds until it starts to gather together to form a dough, and then add enough water to make a malleable dough.

Put the mixture onto a floured board and knead lightly into a firm dough. Add a little more water if the mixture is too dry and then wrap it in clingfilm (plastic wrap) and chill for 30 minutes.

Roll the dough out on to a floured board, quarter of the dough at a time, and cut with a pastry cutter into 48 x 7cm / $2^3/_4$ inch circles (for the bases) and 48 x 5cm/2 inch circles (for the lids). Add little drops of extra water if the dough becomes too dry and crumbly when being rolled out.

Grease and flour 48 non-stick patty tins and line with circles of baking parchment (wax paper). Line the prepared tins with the larger pastry circles.

Fill the pastry with a large teaspoon of mincemeat and cover with the lids. Sprinkle with caster (superfine) sugar and cinnamon and bake for 25 minutes until golden.

Leave the mince pies to cool slightly before easing them out of the tins and onto wire racks.

Store in an airtight container until needed. Warm through before serving and dust with sifted icing (confectioners') sugar.

To make the custard, mix the egg yolks, sugar, cornflour (cornstarch) and ginger syrup in a large mixing bowl. Warm the milk in a non-stick saucepan and then gradually stir into the bowl of eggs. Transfer the mixture back to the saucepan and cook very gently over a low heat, stirring most of the time, until you have a thick and smooth custard. Add the ginger wine. Remove from the heat just as it reaches boiling point – do not boil. Pour into a clean bowl and stir from time to time, as it cools slightly.

Serve in two warm sauceboats with the mince pies or Christmas pudding.

CHAPTER 9

Cold Desserts

Amaretto Tipsy Trifle

A boozy trifle for any time of year. Ideal after a roast for Sunday lunch or at Christmas. You can substitute raspberries with any fruit such as apricots, bananas or blackberries.

Serves 6

100g/3¹/₂oz/²/₃ cup of rice flour

70g/2¹/₂oz/¹/₂ cup of maize flour

3 teaspoons of (GF) baking powder

100g/3¹/₂oz/7 tablespoons of (DF) margarine

100g/3¹/₂oz/1¹/₄ cups of ground almonds

2 large free-range eggs

4 tablespoons of apple juice

1 teaspoon of pure Madagascan vanilla extract

60ml/2fl oz/¹/₄ cup of Amaretto di Saronno liqueur

CUSTARD

3 large free-range egg yolks

1 heaped teaspoon of (GF) cornflour (cornstarch)

1 teaspoon of pure Madagascan vanilla extract

2 tablespoons of Amaretto di Saronno liqueur

240ml/8fl oz/1 cup of soya cream

200ml/7fl oz/³/₄ cup of coconut cream

Some extra Amaretto liqueur

340g/12oz/1 cup of sugar-free raspberry jam (jelly)

2 large bananas, peeled and sliced

255g/9oz/2¹/₄ cups of fresh raspberries

70g/2¹/₂oz/²/₃ cup of (GF/DF) Amaretto di Saronno biscuits (cookies), crumbled

1 litre/1³/₄ pint/1 quart pudding basin and some baking parchment (wax paper), both greased with (DF) margarine

String

Sift the flours and baking powder together in a bowl. In a food processor, mix the margarine, almonds, eggs, juice, vanilla extract and Amaretto until smooth. Quickly blend the flours into this mixture. Scrape into the greased pudding basin. Cover with the greased paper and secure with string around the top, making a handle to remove the basin from the pan later.

Half-fill a saucepan with boiling water and simmer the pudding for 1 hour until firm. Lift the basin out of the pan and leave to cool. Turn out the sponge and cut it into thin slices.

Now make the custard. Mix the egg yolks, cornflour (cornstarch), vanilla extract and Amaretto together with the soya cream and coconut cream. Cook very gently in a non-stick pan, stirring all the time, until it comes to the boil. Immediately remove the pan from the heat and allow to cool, stirring occasionally.

Use a pretty glass bowl and arrange a layer of sponge slices around the base and sides, sprinkle with extra Amaretto di Saronno liqueur. Spread all over with three quarters of the jam (jelly) and then put the bananas on the bottom. Pour over half of the custard. Cover with the remaining sponge and spread the rest of the jam (jelly) over the sponge and top with all the raspberries.

Cover with the remaining custard, sprinkle with the crumbled Amaretto di Saronno biscuits (cookies), and chill until needed.

Lavender Summer Pudding

The lavender fields in the South of France are so beautiful in June. The seemingly endless lines of swaying purple lavender flowers with their heavenly scent inspired this twist on the traditional summer pudding.

Serves 6

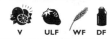

1kg/2.2lbs/6 heaped cups of frozen (thawed) or fresh summer berries such as strawberries, raspberries, blackberries, black and red currants

425ml/15fl oz/scant 2 cups of red vermouth

Juice and zest of 1 small orange

1 tablespoon of fresh lavender flowers, washed in cold water

2 heaped tablespoons of caster (superfine) sugar

1 tablespoon of (WF) cornflour (cornstarch) dissolved in 1 tablespoon of cold water

2 tablespoons of distilled lavender water

1 loaf of (WF) white or a light brown bread

Some little sprigs of fresh lavender for decoration

900ml/1 1/2 pint/4 cup pudding basin

If you are using frozen fruit, let the juices drain into a dish so that you can use them in the recipe. Put any juices with the vermouth, orange juice and zest, lavender flowers and sugar into a non-stick saucepan and bring to the boil. Turn down the heat and simmer until the liquid is reduced by half. Stir in the dissolved cornflour (cornstarch), bring to the boil and simmer for 1 minute. As soon as the sauce is very thick and clear, take the pan off the heat. Remove the sprigs of lavender and discard them.

Stir the lavender water and all the fruit into the thick sauce and leave it to cool. The fruit will inevitably let out more juices, so the sauce must be very thick. If you have any doubts then add a little more dissolved cornflour (cornstarch) and boil up again before adding the lavender water and berries.

Slice the bread very thinly, trim the crusts off and cut the slices diagonally into halves. Line the bottom and sides of the pudding basin with the triangles of bread. When the berry mixture is cold, fill the lined basin with the mixture, then cover the fruit with the remaining bread.

Place a plate directly on top of the bread – it should just fit into the basin and cover the bread completely. Press the plate down with a weight or a heavy can. Put the basin onto a larger plate to catch any overflowing juices, and chill the pudding in the refrigerator for 8–24 hours.

Just before serving, turn the pudding onto a large plate and decorate with sprigs of fresh lavender. If you turn the pudding out too early it might collapse or bulge slightly, so it is better left to the last minute to guarantee perfect results.

Vacherin aux Marrons

If you have had enough of strawberries then this recipe is delicious made with raspberries in the summer or poached, canned pears in the winter.

Serves 8–12

---

4 large free-range egg whites

225g/8oz/1 cup of caster (superfine) sugar

1 teaspoon of pure Madagascan vanilla extract

225g/8oz/2 cups of chopped walnuts

425g/15oz of canned unsweetened chestnut purée

55g/2oz/½ cup of icing (confectioners') sugar, sifted

2 tablespoons of dark rum

2 tablespoons of soya cream, or sufficient to make a spreadable purée

500g/17oz/3½ cups fresh strawberries, washed, hulled and left to dry

30g/1oz of (DF/GF) continental dark chocolate, coarsely grated

Extra icing (confectioners') sugar sifted, to decorate

Draw around 2 dinner plates on 2 sheets of baking parchment (wax paper) and place each sheet on a non-stick baking tray

---

Preheat the oven to 180°C/350°F/Gas mark 4

Whisk the egg whites until they stand in stiff peaks. Whisk in the sugar, a little at a time, until thick and glossy. Fold in the vanilla extract and nuts using a metal spoon.

Lightly spread the mixture over both of the prepared circles of paper.

Bake the meringues in the oven for about 35–45 minutes, or until lightly coloured on top and set inside (unless you are very lucky and have two ovens, I usually swap their positions around at half time, so that they are evenly cooked).

Meanwhile, beat the chestnut purée with the icing (confectioners') sugar, rum and soya cream until it reaches a spreadable consistency.

Slice up the strawberries.

As soon as the vacherin is cold, carefully peel off the paper and place one vacherin on a serving plate. Spread all the chestnut purée on the top of the base and then cover with the strawberries. Cover with the remaining vacherin and decorate the top with the grated chocolate and sifted icing (confectioners') sugar.

Chocolate Profiteroles

Once you can make profiteroles, all sorts of alternatives can be dreamt up. In this recipe the profiteroles are filled with coffee crème patissière and covered in coffee icing, but you could also fill them with (DF) ice-cream and serve with a fruit sauce.

Serves 6 (4 each)

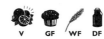

PROFITEROLES

55g/2oz/¹/₄ cup of (DF) margarine
70g/2¹/₂oz/¹/₂ cup of rice flour
2 large free-range eggs
200g/7oz of (DF/GF) plain chocolate
4 tablespoons of freshly brewed espresso coffee
20g/³/₄oz/1¹/₂ tablespoons of (DF) margarine

CRÈME PATISSIÈRE

450ml/15fl oz/scant 2 cups of soya milk
55g/2oz/scant ¹/₄ cup of caster (superfine) sugar
55g/2oz/¹/₃ cup of (GF) cornflour (cornstarch)
2 large free-range egg yolks
4 tablespoons of very strong espresso coffee

Baking parchment (wax paper)

Preheat the oven to 220°C/425°F/Gas mark 7

Mix all the ingredients for the crème patissière in a food processor until smooth, then transfer to a non-stick saucepan.

Cook over medium heat until the custard is thick. Bring to the boil and remove from the heat immediately. Allow the custard to cool slightly, then transfer to a bowl. Cover with baking parchment (wax paper) to prevent a skin forming and chill for 1 hour.

If it is then too firm to spoon or pipe into the profiteroles, add a little more coffee and beat until smooth and manageable.

Make the profiteroles. Heat a pan containing 125ml/4fl oz/¹/₂ cup of water and the 55g/2oz/¹/₄ cup of margarine until boiling. Remove from the heat and tip all the flour into the water. Beat vigorously with a wooden spoon until the mixture leaves the sides of the pan. Add one egg at a time, beating until the dough is smooth and shiny.

Drop 24 teaspoons of dough onto a non-stick baking tray, keeping them about 5cm/2 inches apart. Bake for 25–30 minutes, or until puffy and golden. (Try not to open the oven door until they are ready or they might sink.)

When the profiteroles are ready, remove them from the oven and very quickly pierce them with a sharp knife around the middle. This allows the steam to escape and prevents them from going soggy. Transfer them to a wire rack to cool.

Meanwhile, place the chocolate in a bowl with the coffee and the 20g/³/₄oz/1¹/₂ tablespoons of margarine and melt in the microwave. When melted, stir until smooth and keep to one side.

Slice each cold profiterole across and spoon or pipe in the filling. Close the profiterole and place on a serving plate.

It is traditional to build up the profiteroles into a pyramid shape but they can be arranged however you like. Pour the warm sauce over the tops and serve. The profiteroles can be kept chilled until needed, but serve them on the day of making.

Pineapple Pavlova with Kiwi Sauce

Over the years, I have seen Pavlovas filled with masses of different fruits and creams and they have all been delicious. This one, however, is my favourite because there is a wonderful contrast between the tart kiwi sauce and the sweet, crunchy and marshmallowy meringue.

Serves 8

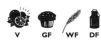

PAVLOVA

285g/10oz/1½ cups of caster (superfine) sugar
1 rounded teaspoon of (GF) cornflour (cornstarch)
5 large free-range egg whites
1 teaspoon of cider or white wine vinegar

FILLING

8 ripe kiwi fruit, peeled, trimmed and quartered
Caster (superfine) sugar to taste

White rum to taste
(DF) vanilla ice-cream
1 medium pineapple, peeled, trimmed, core removed and the flesh cut into bite size cubes

A baking tray lined with a sheet of baking parchment (wax paper)
Draw a circle on the baking parchment (wax paper), around a 23cm/9 inch plate

Preheat the oven to 150°C/300°F/Gas mark 2

Sift the caster (superfine) sugar and cornflour (cornstarch) together into a bowl and set aside. Whisk the egg whites in a large bowl until they form stiff peaks, then fold in the vinegar. Whisk in 50g/2oz/¼ cup of the sugar mixture then, using a metal spoon, fold in the remainder a quarter at a time. Try to let in as much air as possible.

Gently spread the meringue over the circle of paper. Use the back of the spoon to swirl out an indentation in the centre of the meringue and build up the edges higher than the middle. Use a fork to create some peaks around the edge.

Cook the pavlova in the oven for about 25 minutes, or until well risen and a light pinkish-brown. Reduce the heat to 140°C/275°F/Gas mark 1 and cook for another 50 minutes. Turn off the heat but do not open the door. Leave the Pavlova for 2–6 hours inside the oven.

Remove the meringue from the oven and carefully peel away the baking parchment (wax paper). Place the meringue on a serving dish.

Very briefly purée the kiwi fruit in a food processor, but do not use a liquidizer as this results in a discoloured sauce. Add enough sugar to taste and stir in enough rum to make it a perfect pouring consistency. Sieve the sauce to remove the pips and then transfer it to a serving jug.

Fill the pavlova with the ice-cream, then cover with the pineapple and serve immediately with the accompanying sauce.

Marbled Peach Cheesecake

This cheesecake is also delicious made with apricots or nectarines. You can replace the goat's/sheep's yogurt with soya yogurt if necessary, but it is not quite so good.

Serves 8

PEACH PURÉE

255g/9oz/1 1/2 cups ready-to-eat dried peaches
Zest of 1 lemon and the juice of half the lemon
55g/2oz/scant 1/4 cup of caster (superfine) sugar
Juice of 2 oranges
4 tablespoons of Cointreau

THE BASE

55g/2oz/1/2 cup of chopped toasted hazelnuts
100g/3 1/2 oz of ready-made (GF) plain, flavoured
(ie. ginger) or chocolate cookies
55g/2oz/scant 1/4 cup of caster (superfine) sugar
55g/2oz/1/4 cup of (DF) margarine, melted

THE FILLING

3 × 227g/8oz tubs of set sheep's Greek-style yogurt
or goat's yogurt
200g/7oz/1 cup of caster (superfine) sugar
2 large free-range eggs plus 2 large free-range egg
yolks
40g/1 1/2oz/5 tablespoons of rice flour
140ml/5fl oz/2/3 cup of coconut cream
2 fresh and ripe peaches, peeled, stoned (pitted)
and sliced or
425g/15oz canned peach halves in natural juice,
drained and sliced

23cm/9 inch fluted, ovenproof, china quiche dish or
spring-form cake tin

Preheat the oven to 170°C/325°F/Gas mark 3

Place the peaches, lemon zest, sugar and 300ml/10fl oz/1 1/4 cups of water in a pan and bring slowly to the boil. Simmer for about 20 minutes so that the liquid reduces.

When the fruit is soft and mushy, allow it to cool, then liquidize with half the orange juice and half the Cointreau, so that it is very thick.

Make the base by grinding the hazelnuts, cookies and sugar in a food processor until they resemble fine breadcrumbs. Add the melted margarine and process briefly. Press the mixture down into the base of the dish. Bake the base in the oven for 5 minutes.

Beat the yogurt, sugar, eggs, flour and coconut cream together in a bowl and when it is smooth, stir in half of the peach purée to create a marbled effect throughout.

Spoon the mixture over the cooked base and level it off. Arrange the fresh or canned peaches in slices over the top – fan shapes look great.

Bake in the oven for around 50 minutes, or until the cheesecake is firm and dark golden brown. It is a good idea to turn the cheesecake around half way through baking, so that it cooks evenly. Cool completely before refrigerating. Cover and chill until needed.

Add the remaining orange juice and Cointreau to the peach purée. Stir in enough water to make the purée suitable for pouring from a serving jug. Chill the peach purée until needed.

Serve the cheesecake from the dish with the accompanying peach purée.

French Apple Tart

A classic piece of French pâtisserie, which I have tried to make quicker in case time is short between getting home from work and friends coming to dinner.

Serves 10

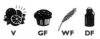

140g/5oz/1 cup of rice flour
140g/5oz/1 cup of maize flour
140g/5oz/²⁄₃ cup of (DF) margarine
55g/2oz/4 tablespoons of caster (superfine) sugar
A pinch of salt
1 large free-range egg
500ml/17fl oz/2 cups of pure and sweetened
   ready-made apple purée

3 large sweet dessert apples, peeled, quartered,
   cored and left in the juice of ¹⁄₂ a small lemon
115g/4oz/¹⁄₃ cup of apricot jam (jelly)

32cm/12¹⁄₂ inch fluted, loose-bottomed tart tin,
   greased and floured

Preheat the oven to 200°C/400°F/Gas mark 6

Combine the flours, margarine, sugar, salt and egg together in a food processor with 2 tablespoons of cold water. Process until it forms a ball of dough.

Put the pastry into the middle of the prepared tin and gently flatten it with floured hands, gently pushing the pastry out until it reaches the sides and then up the fluted sides to the top. Trim the pastry with a knife and discard the trimmings.

Pour the apple purée into the pastry and smooth over. Slice the apple quarters horizontally into wafer thin slices and arrange in overlapping circles in the tart.

Bake the tart for 45 minutes, or until the apples are browned and tender. Keep the tart in the tin while it cools down.

Heat the apricot jam (jelly) in a small bowl in the microwave and spread all over the apples.

Once the tart is cold, remove it carefully from the tin and serve on a plate.

This is delicious with (DF) vanilla ice-cream, if you can not eat crème fraiche.

Redcurrant and Lime Meringue Tarts

These deliciously chewy tarts are easy to transport on picnics, or for summer parties in the garden.
You can use any soft fruit you like for the recipe and in winter, mincemeat is also a delicious option.

Serves 14

PASTRY
200g/7oz/scant 1 1/2 cups of (WF) flour
55g/2oz/1/2 cup of icing (confectioners') sugar
A pinch of salt
100g/3 1/2oz/7 tablespoons of (DF) margarine
1 large free-range egg

FILLING
455g/1lb/2 2/3 cups of redcurrants
200g/7oz/1 cup of caster (superfine) sugar

3 large free-range egg whites
A pinch of salt
Finely grated zest of 2 small limes
1/2 teaspoon of cream of tartar
30g/1oz/scant 1/4 cup of (WF) flour, sifted
1/4 teaspoon of (WF) baking powder
100g/3 1/2oz/1 cup of desiccated (shredded) coconut

2 or more bun trays, greased, floured and lined with
  baking parchment (wax paper) circles

Preheat the oven to 180°C/350°F/Gas mark 4

Make the pastry by combining all the pastry ingredients, except the egg, in a food processor until the mixture resembles breadcrumbs. Add the egg and pulse until the dough comes together into a ball.

Cut the pastry in half and roll out, one half at a time, on a floured surface with a floured rolling pin. Cut our 12 or more circles with a 8 1/2 cm/3 1/4 inch cutter and line each prepared bun tin with the pastry circles.

Divide the redcurrants between the tarts, but do not over fill or they will overflow and become too sticky (if they are large fresh redcurrants then you may not need all the fruit). Sprinkle a little of the sugar over them if the fruit is very sharp.

Make the meringue by whisking the egg whites until stiff in a large bowl with the salt. Gradually beat in all the sugar, then change to a very low speed and add the zest of the limes, followed by the cream of tartar, flour and baking powder. Lastly fold in the coconut.

Place a spoonful of meringue on each tart, keeping the meringue within the boundaries of the pastry so that it doesn't stick to the sides of the tin.

Bake in the oven for about 20–25 minutes, or until the pastry and meringue is golden brown and firm.

Leave the tarts in the tins until they are only just warm. Carefully ease them out of the tins, discard the paper circles and serve the tarts warm or cold.

Strawberry Tarts with Rose Zabaglione

Raspberries are just as delicious as strawberries in these lovely little tarts and very ripe and juicy blackberries in the autumn too. You can always use orange blossom water instead of rosewater for the blackberries.

Makes 16 small tarts

PASTRY
200g/7oz/scant 1½ cups of (WF) flour
55g/2oz/½ cup of icing (confectioners') sugar
A pinch of salt
100g/3½oz/7 tablespoons of (DF) margarine
1 large free-range egg

Variegated lemon balm, to decorate
16-hole bun tray, greased, floured and lined with
   baking parchment (wax paper) circles

FILLING
750g/1lb 10oz/5½ cups of fresh strawberries, hulled
   and wiped clean
340g/12oz/1 generous cup of redcurrant jelly to glaze
   the fruit

ROSE ZABAGLIONE
4 large free-range egg yolks
70g/2½oz/⅓ cup of caster (superfine) sugar
75ml/2½ fl oz/¼ cup of white rum
3 tablespoons of rosewater

Preheat the oven to 180°C/350°F/Gas mark 4

Make the pastry by putting all the pastry ingredients, except the egg, together in the food processor and mixing until it resembles breadcrumbs. Now add the egg and pulse until the dough comes together into a ball.

Cut the pastry in half and roll out each half on a floured surface with a floured rolling pin. Cut out 16 circles with a 8½cm/3¼ inch cutter and line each prepared bun tin with the pastry. Place a circle of baking parchment (wax paper) in each one and secure with some baking beans. Bake blind in the oven for 20 minutes, or until the pastry is golden and crispy.

Remove the tarts from the oven to cool but leave them in the tins. Once they are nearly cold, transfer them to a wire rack.

Cut the strawberries into quarters in order to keep them to an even size and pile plenty of the fruit into each tart.

Use as much or as little jelly as you like to glaze the fruit. Melt the jelly in a small bowl in the microwave and brush each tart with the warm jelly.

Make the zabaglione just before serving. Fill a saucepan a third of the way up with water and bring to the boil. Put the egg yolks and sugar into a large heatproof bowl and beat together with an electric whisk.

Add the rum and rosewater. Place the bowl over the saucepan of simmering water and whisk on high speed until very thick. Serve immediately.

Place a tart on each plate surrounded by a pool of the zabaglione and decorate with a sprig of variegated lemon balm.

Chocolate and Ginger Biscuit Cake

This delicious cake is quick and easy to make. Make sure you have a secret supply of (GF, WF & DF) ginger biscuits or chocolate biscuits in the cupboard, as this makes a great emergency pudding.

Serves 6

V   GF   WF   DF

CRUST
125g/4½oz of (GF/WF/DF) gingernut cookies
55g/2oz/¼ cup of (DF) margarine, melted
55g/2oz/scant ¼ cup of caster (superfine) sugar

FILLING
340g/12oz of (DF/GF) dark chocolate
140g/5oz/⅔ cup of (DF) margarine
240ml/8fl oz/1 cup of soya cream

4 tablespoons of ginger wine, or the drained syrup
   from the stem ginger
2 large free-range eggs, separated
100g/3½oz/½ cup of stem ginger in syrup, drained
   and finely chopped
A little (DF/GF) cocoa powder to dust

24 x 4cm/9½ x 1½-inch-deep ovenproof china or
   glass tart dish, lightly oiled

Preheat the oven to 180°C/350°F/Gas mark 4

Make the crust by mixing the cookies with the margarine and sugar in a food processor until it resembles a loose crumbly mixture.

Press the crumb mixture into the base of the prepared dish, ensuring it is level. Bake in the oven for 10 minutes and then set aside to cool.

Once the base is cold, make the filling by melting the chocolate, margarine, soya cream, ginger wine or syrup in a bowl in the microwave until soft. Remove from the microwave and stir until smooth. Add the egg yolks to the mixture, blend in and then mix in the chopped ginger.

In a separate bowl, whisk the egg whites until they form stiff peaks and fold them gently into the chocolate mixture.

Pour the mixture on to the crust and level off. Chill for 1 hour in the freezer, before transferring to the refrigerator to set.

Cover until needed. Just before serving, dust the biscuit cake with sieved cocoa powder and serve chilled for the best result.

Lemon Tart

This should be baked the day before and kept in the refrigerator, making it an an ideal pudding if you are going to be rushed off your feet on the day of your party.

Serves 8

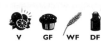

PASTRY

85g/3oz/6 tablespoons of (DF) margarine

45g/1 ¹/₂oz/3 tablespoons of caster (superfine) sugar

Grated zest of 1 lemon

1 large free-range egg

55g/2oz/scant ¹/₂ cup of rice flour

55g/2oz/scant ¹/₂ cup of maize flour

FILLING

3 large free-range eggs

3 large free-range egg yolks

180ml/6fl oz/scant ³/₄ cup of lemon juice

Zest of 1 lemon

200g/7oz/1 cup of caster (superfine) sugar

55g/2oz/¹/₄ cup of (DF) margarine

2 tablespoons of caster (superfine) sugar for sprinkling

8 wafer thin slices of lemon, halved

Extra icing (confectioners') sugar for decoration

24cm/9¹/₂ inch loose-bottomed tart tin, greased and floured

Baking parchment (wax paper) and ceramic baking beans

Preheat the oven to 200°C/400°F/Gas mark 6

Briefly mix the margarine, sugar and grated lemon zest in a food processor. Add the egg and beat for a moment or two. Mix in the flours until it comes together into a dough. Shape the pastry into a ball, wrap in clingfilm (plastic wrap) and chill for 1 hour.

Roll out the dough on a floured surface to the shape of the tin. Transfer the pastry to the tin and press into the tin with floured fingers. Trim the edges and prick all over the base of the pastry with a fork.

Line the pastry with the baking parchment (wax paper), cover with ceramic beans and bake for 15 minutes. Carefully remove the ceramic beans and baking parchment (wax paper) and cook the pastry in the oven for a further 5 minutes. Set aside to cool.

Now make the filling in a food processor. Beat the 3 whole eggs with the 3 extra yolks, lemon juice and zest, and sugar. Transfer to a non-stick saucepan and cook gently over medium heat. Stir frequently and do not allow it to boil. When the mixture is thick, remove from the heat, add the margarine and stir until it has melted.

Pour the filling into the pastry shell and chill in the refrigerator for 12 hours.

A couple of hours before serving the lemon tart, turn the grill (broiler) on to very hot. Sprinkle the extra sugar over the lemon filling and decorate with the lemon slices. Grill (broil) for about 6–8 minutes until the tart is browned but not scorched.

Chill the tart again until needed. To serve, slide the base off the tin onto a serving dish and decorate the tart with a sprinkling of extra sifted icing (confectioners') sugar.

Chocolate Sachetorte

This is a dreamy Viennese cake, which is eaten in cafés all over the city with steaming cups of coffee or hot chocolate.

Serves 8

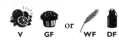

310g/11oz of (DF/GF) dark chocolate and a little extra chocolate for decoration

170g/6oz/³⁄4 cup of (DF) margarine

115g/4oz/¹⁄2 cup plus 1 tablespoon of caster (superfine) sugar

100g/3¹⁄2 oz/1¹⁄4 cups of ground almonds

4 large free-range eggs, separated

55g/2oz/1 cup of 100% pure (WF) rye or (GF) corn breadcrumbs

2 tablespoon of sugar-free apricot or raspberry jam (jelly)

55g/2oz/¹⁄2 cup of icing (confectioners') sugar

2 tablespoons of black coffee

23cm/9 inch spring-form cake tin, greased with (DF) margarine and lined with baking parchment (wax paper)

Preheat the oven to 180°C/350°F/Gas mark 4

Break half the chocolate into a bowl, microwave it until just melting and then stir until smooth.
Cream 115g/4oz/¹⁄2 cup of the margarine and the sugar together in a bowl. Stir in the almonds, egg yolks and breadcrumbs, then fold in the melted chocolate and beat well.
Whisk the egg whites until stiff and then fold half at a time into the chocolate mixture. Pour into the prepared cake tin. Bake the cake for 40 minutes until firm to the touch. Allow to cool for 45 minutes and then turn out onto a serving plate. Brush the cake with the jam (jelly).
Melt the remaining chocolate and margarine together in a bowl in the microwave. Stir and sift in the icing (confectioners') sugar and then beat in the black coffee. Leave to stand for 5 minutes. Spread the icing all over the cake. Coarsely grate some extra chocolate on top of the cake and serve chilled.

Raspberry Gallette

Making pastry on a marble board keeps everything lovely and cool and gives excellent results.
If you are in a hurry, you can fill the gallette with suitable (DF) vanilla ice-cream and raspberries
and serve before it melts!

Serves 8

225g/8oz/1²/₃ cups of rice flour, sifted
35g/1¼oz/¹/₃ cup of ground almonds
50g/1³/₄oz/¹/₃ cup of icing (confectioners') sugar
115g/4oz/¹/₂ cup of (DF) margarine
The grated rind of 1 orange
2 large free-range egg yolks
1 teaspoon of orange flower water

CRÈME PATISSIERE
3 large free-range egg yolks
40g/1¹/₂oz/3 tablespoons of caster (superfine) sugar
¹/₂ teaspoon of almond essence
1 tablespoon of (GF) cornflour (cornstarch)
240ml/8fl oz/1 cup of soya milk

15g/¹/₂oz/1 tablespoon of (DF) margarine
Enough coconut cream to make the crème
 spreadable

500g/17oz/4 cups of fresh raspberries
Icing (confectioners') sugar to dust
Mint leaves and spare raspberries to decorate

COULIS
500g/17oz/4 cups of mixed red summer fruit
The juice of ¹/₂ a lemon
Rum and water
Icing (confectioners') sugar, optional

Preheat the oven to 180°C/350°F/Gas mark 4

Place the flour, almonds, sugar, margarine and orange rind into a food processor and blend until it resembles fine breadcrumbs. Mix in the egg yolks and orange flower water.

Wrap the dough in clingfilm (plastic wrap) and chill for 1 hour. Divide the pastry in half and roll it out thinly. Use a 23cm/9 inch plate as a template to cut out 2 circles and place on a baking sheet. Mark each circle into 8 wedges, scored almost through the pastry. Bake for 20 minutes until golden. Transfer to a wire rack to cool.

Make the crème patissiere. Put the egg yolks, sugar, almond essence and flour in a bowl and mix. Gradually beat in the milk and then transfer the mixture to a non-stick saucepan. Gently cook over a low heat, bringing it slowly to the boil. Keep stirring all the time until it is smooth and thick. Transfer to a bowl and dot with margarine to stop a skin forming. When cold, mix in the coconut cream until spreadable. Spread the cream all over the pastry circles and set on a plate. Cover with raspberries and then the top layer of pastry. Dust with icing (confectioners') sugar and decorate the plate with a few mint leaves and raspberries.

Make the coulis. Purée the fruit with the lemon juice and enough rum/water to make a thick sauce – sweeten to taste if necessary with the sugar. Serve the coulis with the gallette.

Strawberry Shortcake

English strawberries are so wonderful in the summer and this is such an English-style pudding!

Serves 6

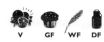

30g/1oz/2 tablespoons of sugar
130g/4¹/₂oz/generous ³/₄ cup of rice flour
100g/3¹/₂oz/²/₃ cup of millet flour
1 tablespoon of (GF) baking powder
¹/₄ teaspoon of salt
55g/2oz/¹/₄ cup of (DF) margarine
3 teaspoons of rosewater
5 tablespoons of natural soya yogurt (or goat's yogurt, which is not DF), beaten with 3 large eggs

4 tablespoons of redcurrant jelly, warmed in a saucepan
750ml/25fl oz/3 cups of (DF) vanilla ice-cream
500g/17oz/3¹/₂ cups of strawberries, rinsed thoroughly and sliced

23cm/9 inch round cake tin, greased, floured and lined with baking parchment (wax paper)

Preheat the oven to 200°C/400°F/Gas mark 6

Sift the dry ingredients together in a bowl and rub (cut) in the margarine until it resembles breadcrumbs. Lightly mix the rosewater, yogurt and eggs together and blend into the dry ingredients.
Scrape the mixture into the prepared cake tin and bake for about 20 minutes, or until golden brown. Cool and then split open the shortcake with a long knife.
Gently heat the redcurrant jelly in a saucepan until melted and then keep warm.
Put the shortcake base on a plate and brush with half of the warm redcurrant jelly. When the shortcake is cold, spoon on softened vanilla ice-cream and cover with half of the strawberries.
Place the remaining cake on top, add the rest of the strawberries and brush with the warm jelly to glaze. Serve immediately.

Sherry Cake and Baked Figs

A splash of Sherry or Marsala transforms this cake into an exciting delicacy. Both these fortified wines bring the full taste sensation of sun-baked, ripe Mediterranean figs bursting in your mouth as you bite into them.

Serves 6

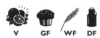

CAKE

70g/2¹/₂oz/¹/₂ cup of potato flour
100g/3¹/₂oz/²/₃ cup of maize flour
100g/3¹/₂oz/²/₃ cup of rice flour
2 teaspoons of (GF) baking powder
A pinch of salt
225ml/7¹/₂ fl oz/generous ³/₄ cup of light
  sunflower oil
225g/8oz/1 generous cup of caster (superfine) sugar
4 large free-range eggs
130g/4¹/₂oz/1¹/₂ cups of ground almonds
Grated zest of 1 lemon
125ml/4fl oz/¹/₂ cup of aged Amontillado dry sherry
Icing (confectioners') sugar to decorate

FIGS

12 ripe, but firm, figs
Juice of 1 large orange
³/₄ teaspoon of pure Madagascan vanilla extract
1 teaspoon of (GF) mixed (pie) spice
A little grated nutmeg
3 tablespoons of Marsala
3 tablespoons of runny honey

20cm/8 inch non-stick cake tin, greased and dusted
  with extra flour

Preheat the oven to 180°C/350°F/Gas mark 4

Sift the flours, baking powder and salt into a large bowl. In another bowl, whisk the oil with the sugar and beat in the eggs, one at a time, until thick and creamy.
Gently fold the egg mixture into the flours. Carefully add the almonds, lemon zest and sherry, and spoon the cake mixture into the prepared tin.
Bake for 1 hour, or until an inserted skewer comes out clean.
Allow the cake to cool, then turn out onto a wire rack and leave until cold.
Wash the figs and place them in an ovenproof dish with the orange juice, vanilla extract, spices and Marsala. Pour the honey over the figs and bake for 35 minutes or until soft and glazed. Put the cake on a plate and sprinkle with icing (confectioners') sugar. Serve the figs warm or cold with the cake.

Mocha Mousse Cake

The base for this cake can also be made into delicious cookies. Dust them with extra sugar and serve with (DF) ice-cream or just with freshly brewed coffee for a special treat.

Serves 6–8

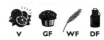

SHORTBREAD CRUST

100g/3½oz/7 tablespoons of (DF) margarine

5 tablespoons of caster (superfine) sugar

1 teaspoon of pure Madagascan vanilla extract

100g/3½oz/⅔ cup of rice flour

5 tablespoons of unsweetened (DF/GF) cocoa powder

¼ teaspoon of salt

100g/3½oz/1 generous cup of ground almonds

2 tablespoons of caster (superfine) sugar

55g/2oz/¼ cup of melted (DF) margarine

MOCHA MOUSSE

100g/3½oz of (DF/GF) dark continental chocolate

4 large free-range egg yolks

100g/3½oz/½ cup of caster (superfine) sugar

140ml/5fl oz/⅔ cup of strong freshly brewed, hot black coffee

11.7g/½oz sachet (US 1 tablespoon) powdered gelatine dissolved in 60ml/2fl oz/¼ cup of boiling water, or vegetarian equivalent

3 large free-range egg whites

8–16 fresh coffee beans for decoration and a little extra (DF/GF) cocoa powder

A deep-sided 23cm/9 inch china or glass tart or flan dish, lightly oiled

---

Preheat the oven to 180°C/350°F/Gas mark 4

Make the shortbread crust first. Mix together the margarine, sugar and vanilla extract until pale and creamy, in either a bowl or a food processor. Sift together the flour, cocoa and salt onto a plate. Add the dry ingredients to the margarine mixture and beat together until the dough forms into a ball. Wrap the dough in clingfilm (plastic wrap) and chill for 30 minutes.

On a lightly oiled surface, roll out the dough to 1.25cm/½-inch thick and slide it on to a non-stick baking tray. Bake it in the oven for 25–35 minutes, but do not let the crust blacken around the edges. (Alternatively, if you are making cookies, cut out 5cm/2 inch circles instead and transfer them to a non-stick baking tray, leaving plenty of room for them to spread. Bake the cookies for 20–25 minutes or until firm to touch. Cool on a wire rack.)

When the shortbread crust has cooled down, break it up into pieces and allow it to get cold. Process the shortbread crust briefly in a food processor until it resembles breadcrumbs. Quickly add the almonds, 2 tablespoons of caster (superfine) sugar and the melted margarine, and mix for a second or two.

Pack the shortbread mixture into the prepared dish, press down firmly and then place in the refrigerator to cool.

Meanwhile, melt the chocolate in a large bowl in the microwave until just soft and then stir until smooth. Beat the egg yolks in a food processor with the caster (superfine) sugar until pale and smooth. Pour in the hot coffee and process again. Pour in the melted gelatine and riefly process again. Stir the coffee mixture into the bowl of chocolate until well blended. Leave the mousse to cool in the refrigerator for 20 minutes.

Put the egg whites in a large bowl, beat until stiff and fold into the mousse mixture using a metal spoon.

Pour the mousse over the biscuit base, level off and chill for about 3 hours or until set. Decorate with coffee beans or (DF) chocolate-coated coffee beans and dust with sifted cocoa powder.

Rosewater Angel Cake with Berries

This happens to be a low-fat cake, so it is ideal for weight-watching dinner guests. You can use any mixture of fruit you like to suit whatever is in season.

Serves 8–12

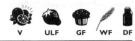

CAKE

125g/4½oz/generous ¾ cup of rice flour, sifted

185g/6½oz/scant 1 cup of caster (superfine) sugar

A pinch of salt

7 large free-range egg whites

2 teaspoons of cream of tartar

1 tablespoon of rosewater

FILLING AND SAUCE

Plenty of fresh soft fruits such as strawberries, blackberries, blueberries, raspberries, stoned (pitted) cherries or currants

White rum

Caster (superfine) sugar to taste

(I have left the quantities optional so that you can use this recipe for a small party of 6 guests or increase the amount of filling and sauce for the maximum of 12 guests)

A large, deep, non-stick ring baking tin or a large, deep, non-stick Kugelhopf tin

---

Preheat the oven to 180°C/350°F/Gas mark 4

Make the cake first. Sift together the flour, 7 tablespoons of the sugar and the salt in a bowl and set aside. In another larger bowl, whisk the egg whites at low speed for 1 minute, or until they are thick and foamy. Add the cream of tartar and increase the speed to medium.

Slowly sprinkle 2 more tablespoons of sugar into the egg whites and beat them until they form soft peaks. Add the rosewater and fold in the remaining sugar, followed by the sifted flour mixture.

Pour the cake mixture into the tin and bake in the oven for about 40 minutes, or until an inserted skewer comes out clean. It should be golden and firm to touch.

Leave the cake to cool in the tin for 20 minutes, after which time the cake should come have away from the sides of the tin. Ease the cake out and turn it onto a large serving plate.

Fill the centre of the cake with as many berries as you like, so that it looks pretty. Keep the rest to make the sauce. Put plenty of berries, some rum and a little sugar into the food processor and pulse to a purée. Adjust the sweetness and the consistency to suit your taste with extra sugar, water and rum. Sieve the sauce and discard all the pips and skins.

The sauce should be just runny enough to spoon over the cake and trickle a little bit down the sides of the cake but not too runny otherwise it will trickle away!

Spoon the sauce decoratively over the sponge ring only, not on the fruit filling.

Serve the rest of the sauce in a pretty jug to accompany the pudding.

Cherry Chocolate Torte

Another blissful combination – cherries, brandy and chocolate! Here it is taken from the past, a Black Forest Gâteau to a trendy modern style of cooking, a torte. Serve with lashings of crème fraîche (not DF) or (DF) vanilla ice-cream.

Serves 6–8

BASE
155g/5½oz/1⅓ cups of (GF) ratafias (almond macaroon cookies)
2 tablespoons of (DF/GF) cocoa powder
55g/2oz/¼ cup of (DF) margarine, melted

CAKE
The same weight of 2 large free-range eggs (in their shells), caster (superfine) sugar
(DF) margarine and rice flour
3 tablespoons of (DF/GF) cocoa powder
3 tablespoons of cherry/brandy liqueur or good quality brandy

1 teaspoon of (GF) baking powder
100g/3½oz/1¼ cups of glacé cherries halved and soaked in brandy for 24 hours if possible, or a small jar of cherries in brandy, drained but brandy retained
85g/3oz/¾ cup of pine nuts
Extra caster (superfine) sugar for sprinkling

23cm/9 inch round loose-bottomed, spring-form cake tin, lined with baking parchment (wax paper)

Preheat the oven to 180°C/350°F/Gas mark 4

Process the ratafias in the food processor until they resemble breadcrumbs. Add the cocoa and melted margarine and mix well. Transfer to the prepared dish and press down firmly to form an even base. Bake in the oven for 5 minutes.

First weigh the eggs, then weigh exactly the same weight of sugar, followed by the margarine and then the flour. Beat the sugar and margarine together until light and fluffy in a food processor. Beat in the cocoa powder and then the eggs, one at a time. Add the cherry/brandy liqueur or brandy, briefly blend in the flour and quickly stir in the baking powder.

Gently stir in the cherries, then spoon the mixture into the prepared cake tin. Carefully level off the cake, scatter the pine nuts over it and sprinkle with a little extra sugar.

Bake the cake in the oven for 35 minutes, or until the nuts are golden and the cake is firm to touch.

Allow the cake cool down in the tin before easing it out and removing the baking parchment (wax paper). Place the cake on a plate and serve warm or cold.

Banana and Coffee Roulade

Roulades are one of those fun things that look great but are so simple to make. As this one is not filled with cream it will keep in the refrigerator for 24 hours but it must be sealed completely in clingfilm (plastic wrap) otherwise the bananas will go brown.

Serves 8

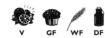

ROULADE
100g/3¹/₂oz/²/₃ cup of rice flour
¹/₂ teaspoon of (GF) baking powder
¹/₂ teaspoon of bicarbonate of soda (baking soda)
A pinch of salt
1 large ripe banana, mashed
2 tablespoons of coconut cream
¹/₂ teaspoon of pure Madagascan vanilla extract
1 tablespoon of white rum
85g/3oz/6 tablespoons of (DF) margarine
100g/3¹/₂oz/¹/₂ cup of caster (superfine) sugar
1 large free-range egg, lightly beaten

FILLING AND DECORATION
30g/1oz/¹/₄ cup of chopped and toasted hazelnuts, for decoration
1 tablespoon of good instant coffee dissolved in 1 tablespoon of boiling water
1 tablespoon of white rum
100g/3¹/₂oz/7 tablespoons of (DF) margarine
200g/7oz/1¹/₂ cups of icing (confectioners') sugar
1–2 ripe small bananas, finely sliced and tossed in another tablespoon of rum (or ¹/₂ a tablespoon of lemon juice if you prefer)
Icing (confectioners') sugar, sifted for decoration

A roulade or Swiss roll tin, lined with baking parchment (wax paper)

Preheat the oven to 180°C/350°F/Gas mark 4

Make the roulade. Sift together the flour, baking powder, bicarbonate of soda (baking soda) and salt. In another bowl, mix together the banana, coconut cream, vanilla and rum.
Beat the margarine and sugar in a food processor until pale and fluffy. Slowly add the egg and then beat for about 30 seconds. Scrape the mixture into the mashed banana, mix briefly and then fold in the flour mixture.
Lightly spread the mixture in the roulade tin and bake in the oven for 15–20 minutes, or until firm to touch and golden.
Leave the roulade to cool for a couple of minutes and then turn it on to a sheet of baking parchment (wax paper) sprinkled all over with the chopped toasted hazelnuts.
Quickly peel off the baking parchment (wax paper) used during cooking and trim the edges of the roulade with a sharp knife (this stops the edges going hard, making it easier to roll up).
Cover with a clean but damp (with cold water) tea towel and set aside until cold. Make the filling in the food processor by beating the dissolved coffee and rum with the margarine and icing (confectioners') sugar until it is smooth and light.

Have the bananas ready and then spread the coffee filling all over the roulade and cover it with the sliced bananas.

Quickly roll the roulade into a log shape and slide on to a long serving dish. Sprinkle over any nuts that have been left behind and then sift over the icing (confectioners') sugar. Serve or chill until needed.

Chestnut and Chocolate Roulade

This is a quick and easy Christmas pudding to make. You can transform it into a Yule log by covering it with chocolate icing, dusting it with icing (confectioners') sugar and adding a festive spring of holly.

Serves 6

V   GF   WF   DF

5 large free-range eggs, separated

170g/6oz/generous ¾ cup of caster (superfine) sugar

140g/5oz of (DF/GF) dark chocolate

3 tablespoons of cold water

½ teaspoon of pure Madagascan vanilla extract

225g/8oz/1 cup of unsweetened chestnut purée

240g/8½oz/1¼ cups of whole chestnuts, drained and roughly chopped

2 tablespoons of brandy, or rum, or fresh black coffee

2 tablespoons of coconut cream

(DF/GF) cocoa powder (or grated [DF/GF] dark chocolate), to dust

A large roulade tin, greased and lined with baking parchment (wax paper)

Preheat the oven to 180°C/350°F/Gas mark 4

Beat the egg yolks in a bowl with the sugar until pale and fluffy. Melt the chocolate in a bowl set over boiling water in the microwave. Stir the chocolate into the egg yolks. Add the cold water and vanilla extract.

Whisk the egg whites until soft peaks are formed and then fold into the chocolate mixture. Spread over the tray, leaving a 2.5cm/1 inch border all round.

Bake until firm and spongy, about 15 minutes.

Set the roulade tin on a wire rack and cover with a clean damp cloth until cold.

Remove the cloth and loosen the paper. Dust another sheet of baking parchment (wax paper) with cocoa and turn the roulade onto it. Peel off the paper. Blend together the chestnut purée, brandy, rum or coffee and coconut cream until smooth and spreadable. Mix in the chopped chestnuts and spread all over the roulade.

Roll up the roulade using the paper beneath it to guide you and serve decorated with extra cocoa or grated chocolate.

Coconut Rice Moulds with Passion Fruit Sauce

This is an exotic pudding, ideal after an Asian or Indian main course. You can substitute this sauce for mango, apricot or any seasonal soft berries that purée well.

Serves 6

V · GF · WF · DF

115g/4oz/²/₃ cup of pudding rice
400ml/14fl oz/1¹/₂ cups of water
400ml/14fl oz/1¹/₂ cups of coconut milk
20g/³/₄oz/1¹/₂ tablespoons of caster (superfine) sugar
11.7g/¹/₂oz sachet (US 1 tablespoon) of powdered gelatine or vegetarian equivalent
200ml/7fl oz/³/₄ cup of coconut cream
2 egg whites with a pinch of salt
Fresh mint leaves to decorate

SAUCE
The juice of 1 lemon
4 passion fruit, halved and scooped out
1 large ripe mango, peeled, sliced and puréed

6 ramekins
Clingfilm (plastic wrap)

Put the rice and water into a large saucepan, bring to the boil and cook gently for 10 minutes.

Add the coconut milk and sugar and simmer for another 35 minutes until it is soft, thick and creamy. Stir from time to time to prevent the rice sticking to the pan.

Prepare the gelatine by dissolving it in 90ml/3fl oz/¹/₃ cup of boiling water and mixing until it is clear. Stir the gelatine into the rice and fold in the coconut cream. Beat the egg whites and gently fold in with a metal spoon.

Now line 6 ramekins with clingfilm (plastic wrap). Spoon the rice pudding into them and smooth over the surfaces. Chill for about 4 hours until set.

Make the passion fruit sauce by mixing the lemon juice and passion fruit pulp with the mango purée and a little extra water until it is the right consistency. Chill until needed.

To serve, turn the rice puddings out onto serving plates and remove the clingfilm (plastic wrap). Pour some of the sauce over and around them and decorate with a sprig of fresh mint.

Carpaccio of Fresh Pineapple with Mint Sauce

The further into the south of France we drove on our honeymoon, the hotter the weather became and so we could enjoy candle lit dinners on the terrace overlooking the gardens and mountains. We did find that higher temperatures put us off very rich puddings, so here is a light, fat-free one, which we very much enjoyed in a superb Château in Provence.

Serves 8

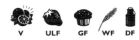

1 large, ripe pineapple, trimmed and peeled

A handful of fresh coriander (cilantro) leaves

Grated zest and juice of 2 fresh limes

1 heaped tablespoon of finely grated root ginger

4 handfuls of fresh mint leaves

2 tablespoons of white rum

240ml/8fl oz/1 cup of unsweetened pineapple juice

Fresh sprigs of little mint leaves to decorate

Slice the pineapple into wafer thin slices using an extremely sharp, long knife. Please do this slowly and carefully! Then, with a small knife, remove the inner core from each slice and discard it.

Arrange the pineapple into rows over a white plate or a glass dish.

Put the coriander (cilantro) leaves, lime juice and zest, grated root ginger, mint leaves, rum and pineapple juice into a food processor. Mix very briefly, so that it has the consistency of a ready-made mint sauce.

Spoon the sauce over the pineapple and serve immediately for ultimate freshness.

Decorate with the extra mint leaves.

Clementine and Orange Jelly

English jelly dates back to the 14th century, and became grander and more elaborate over the centuries. Blancmanges evolved and beautiful gleaming copper and china jelly moulds of every shape and size hung in kitchens until the 1960s, when sadly we 'progressed' to mass-produced jellies.

Serves 4

The juice of 6 large juicy oranges

60ml/2fl oz/¼ cup of Cointreau, orange liqueur (or clementine juice for children)

11.7g/½oz sachet (US 1 tablespoon) of powdered gelatine or vegetarian equivalent, dissolved according to instructions on the packet

310g/11oz/1½ cups of fresh, seedless clementines, peeled, pith removed and segments chopped (canned fruit is fine, just drain the juices)

A few spare segments of clementines and fresh mint to decorate

---

Mix the orange juice with the Cointreau in a bowl and vigorously stir in the gelatine as soon as it has dissolved. Add the chopped clementines and chill for 1 hour, before giving it a thoroughly good stir to distribute the clementines more evenly.

Pour the jelly into glasses or individual tin moulds and chill for 4 hours, or until set.

When the jellies are set, decorate them in the glasses with spare clementines and fresh mint leaves. Alternatively, dip the moulds into boiling water for a few seconds and turn out the jellies on to small plates and decorate around the jelly.

For children, omit the liqueur and mint leaves and make the jellies in pretty paper cups.

Cranberry and Wine Jelly with Grapes

Mix red and white grapes for a pretty effect in this dish, or choose any fruit in season, which can be fresh or poached and then served around the jellies.

Serves 4–6

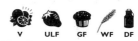

V   ULF   GF   WF   DF

300ml/10fl oz/1¼ cups of red wine

140g/5oz/¾ cup of caster (superfine) sugar

Zest of 1 orange

1 teaspoon of (GF) mixed (pie) spice

1 sprig of rosemary

600ml/20fl oz/2½ cups of cranberry juice

1½ sachets (17g/¾oz/US 1½ tablespoons) of powdered gelatine or vegetarian equivalent

A fresh bunch of seedless grapes, trimmed, skinned and halved

2–3 tablespoons of redcurrant jelly

A little red wine or port

Juice of 1 large orange

4–6 ramekin dishes or tin jelly moulds, lightly brushed with oil

---

Stir the wine, sugar, orange zest, mixed (pie) spice and rosemary together in a saucepan over medium heat to gently dissolve the sugar. Bring the mixture up to the boil and boil for 5 minutes. Remove the pan from the heat, add the cranberry juice and allow the mixture to infuse for 5 minutes.

Place the saucepan back onto medium heat and bring the cranberry and wine mixture to the boil. Boil for 5 minutes, then remove from the heat and quickly stir in the gelatine. Stir from time to time until the gelatine has dissolved.

Sieve the jelly into a good pouring jug and then pour the wine jelly into the prepared ramekins. Leave the jellies to set for at least 4 hours or until firm enough to turn out.

Meanwhile, prepare as many of the grapes as you think you will need for 4 or 6 guests and put them in a bowl.

Dissolve the redcurrant jelly with the orange juice and a little extra wine or port and bring it to the boil. Adjust the consistency with more liquid or jelly if necessary – it should be just runny enough to coat the grapes. Quickly remove it from the heat and blend thoroughly until smooth.

Pour it over the grapes, cool, then cover and leave it at room temperature until ready to serve.

Turn out the jellies onto plates and spoon the grapes with a little of the liquid around each jelly. Serve straight away.

Summer Fruit Mousse

This is a light and colourful pudding that can be made with frozen fruit throughout the year.

Serves 8

500g/17oz/3 cups of mixed summer fruits
    (frozen or fresh)
100g/3½oz/½ cup of caster (superfine) sugar
The grated rind and juice of 1 lemon
2 tablespoons of gelatine, soaked in 3 tablespoons
    of boiling water until dissolved and clear, or
    vegetarian equivalent
200ml/7fl oz/¾ cup of coconut cream

200ml/7fl oz/¾ cup of soya cream
2 egg whites

FOR DECORATION

1 egg white
115g/4oz/⅔ cup of fresh summer berries
Caster (superfine) sugar

Put the fruit in a saucepan with the sugar, lemon rind and juice. Cook for 5 minutes or until just soft. Add the gelatine and remove from the heat. Sieve into a bowl and leave to cool.

When cool, place the fruit mixture in the refrigerator until it begins to set. Fold in the coconut cream and soya cream.

Whisk the egg whites until stiff and then fold into the mousse with a metal spoon. Spoon this into a pretty glass bowl and smooth over. Chill until set.

Decorate at the last minute. Lightly whisk the egg white. Discard half of it. Dip the fresh fruit in the remaining egg white and then coat with sugar. Arrange on top of the mousse and serve.

Orange Mousse with Almonds

This is more of an exotic orange custard than a mousse. It is delicious served in little ramekins and enjoyed with tiny almond cookies.

Serves 4–6

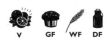

115g/4oz/¹/₂ cup plus 1 tablespoon caster (superfine) sugar

4 large free-range egg yolks

1 large free-range egg

3 tablespoons of pale dry sherry

2 heaped tablespoons of ground almonds

Zest from 1 large or 2 small oranges

300ml/10fl oz/1¹/₄ cups of freshly squeezed orange juice

11.7g/¹/₂oz sachet (US 1 tablespoon) of powdered gelatine, dissolved in 100ml/3fl oz/¹/₃ cup of boiling water, or vegetarian equivalent

1 tablespoon of toasted almond slivers

Beat the sugar, egg yolks and whole egg in a food processor until pale and creamy. Briefly blend in the sherry, ground almonds and orange zest. Transfer the mixture to a large bowl.

Microwave the orange juice until boiling and frothy and then whisk it into the egg mixture at full speed on an electric mixer. Pour in the prepared gelatine, whisking all the time to distribute it evenly.

Pour the mixture into a small soufflé dish or 4–6 ramekins. Leave the mousse to set in the freezer for about 40 minutes, then transfer to the refrigerator for at least 3 hours or until firm. Decorate the mousse with the almond slivers and serve chilled.

Chocolate and Pistachio Bavarois with Orange Sherry Sauce

This is extremely rich, so you can use smaller tin moulds and serve 8 to 10 guests instead. There is plenty of sauce to allow for this!

Serves 6

V   GF   WF   DF

BAVAROIS

255g/9oz of (DF/GF) dark continental chocolate
140g/5oz/²/₃ cup of (DF) margarine
4 large free-range eggs
55g/2oz/scant ¼ cup of caster (superfine) sugar
100g/3½oz/¾ cup of peeled pistachio nuts
A pinch of salt

6 ramekins brushed with sunflower oil and lined with
   a circle of baking parchment (wax paper)

ORANGE SHERRY SAUCE

4 free-range eggs, beaten
200g/7oz/1 cup of caster (superfine) sugar
Grated zest of 1 orange
140ml/5fl oz/²/₃ cup of fresh orange juice
55g/2oz/¼ cup of (DF) margarine, cut into small
   pieces
60ml/2fl oz/¼ cup of pale dry sherry or Marsala

1–2 oranges, pith and pips removed and cut into
   segments for decoration or poached, sliced
   kumquats or fresh physalis fruit (Cape
   gooseberries), and (DF) cream, to decorate

Melt the chocolate with the margarine in a large bowl in the microwave until just soft. Stir the mixture until smooth.

Separate the eggs and put the whites in a very large bowl. Place the yolks and the sugar in a food processor and beat until thick and creamy. Stir this into the chocolate mixture, followed by the nuts.

Beat the egg whites and salt together until soft peaks form. Fold the egg whites into the chocolate mixture using a metal spoon, then divide the mixture between the prepared ramekins.

Cover with clingfilm (plastic wrap) and chill for at least 4 hours, or until firmly set.

Meanwhile, make the sauce. Put all the ingredients, except the margarine and sherry, into a food processor and beat for a few seconds.

Transfer the mixture into a non-stick saucepan and cook over low heat until the mixture thickens to a custard. Keep stirring so that it does not stick to the pan – do not boil the custard or it will separate. Quickly beat in the margarine and sherry. Transfer to a bowl and allow to cool, then cover and chill until needed.

To serve, peel the clingfilm (plastic wrap) off the puddings, dip the ramekins briefly in hot water to loosen the bavarois, then turn them out on to the centre of each plate, pour the orange and sherry sauce around each one and decorate with a couple of orange segments, poached kumquats or fresh physalis fruit (Cape gooseberries) with their wings peeled back. Swirl little drops of (DF) cream into the sauce if desired.

Mango Passion Mousse

This feather light mousse, which is covered with glistening pools of passion fruit, is ideal for a large buffet or party at any time of the year.

Serves 12–14

V GF WF DF

Seeds from 10 cardamom pods

6 large free-range egg yolks

2 tablespoons of caster (superfine) sugar

240ml/8fl oz/1 cup of soya cream

200ml/7fl oz/³⁄₄ cup of coconut cream

3 tablespoons of Cointreau

2 medium (approximately 600g/1lb 5oz each) ripe mangoes, peeled and the flesh roughly chopped

1 freshly squeezed orange

Juice of 1 lemon

1¹⁄₂ sachets (17g/³⁄₄oz/US 1¹⁄₂ tablespoons) powdered gelatine, dissolved in 60ml/2fl oz/¹⁄₄ cup of boiling water and stirred until dissolved, or vegetarian equivalent

3 large free-range egg whites

5 large ripe passion fruit, halved and seeds and juices scooped out and used for decoration

Put the cardamom seeds into a non-stick saucepan with the egg yolks and sugar and beat with a wooden spoon. Gradually add the soya cream, then the coconut cream. Cook the mixture over a low heat until it thickens and comes almost to boiling point, stirring constantly. Remove from the heat and continue to stir.

Add the Cointreau and leave the custard to cool in a clean bowl, stirring occasionally.

Purée the mango and fruit juices together in a food processor until smooth, then stir the purée into the custard.

As soon as the mixture is a little cooler, stir in the dissolved gelatine. Set aside until the mixture is cold.

Whisk the egg whites in a separate bowl until they form stiff peaks. Add a little of the custard to the whisked egg whites and fold in gently. Quickly fold the egg white mixture into the remaining custard using a metal spoon and transfer to a large glass serving bowl. Level off the top and freeze for 40 minutes, to help it set quickly.

Remove the mousse from the freezer and cover with clingfilm (plastic wrap). Chill in the refrigerator for 4 hours or until it is firm and set.

Decorate the mousse by sprinkling spoonfuls of passion fruit over the surface. Serve the mousse chilled.

Classic Chocolate Mousse

As light as a cloud and as popular now as it was 20 years ago, this classic French mousse can not be changed because it is utterly perfect.

Serves 6

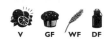

225g/8oz of (DF/GF) dark continental chocolate

15g/¹/₂oz/1 tablespoon of (DF) margarine

1 tablespoon of Cognac or brandy

4 large free-range eggs, separated

6 ramekins

Break the chocolate into small pieces, place in a large bowl with 4 tablespoons of water and melt in the microwave. Stir in the margarine and Cognac and microwave very briefly. Now stir in the egg yolks.

In another bowl, whisk the egg whites until they are stiff and forming firm peaks. Now fold the egg whites into the chocolate mixture using a metal spoon. Gently spoon the mousse mixture into each ramekin and carefully level off.

Cover each mousse with clingfilm (plastic wrap) and chill them for several hours or until they are firmly set.

Remove the clingfilm (plastic wrap) and serve each ramekin on a little plate with a couple of tiny (GF & DF) cookies.

Elderflower and Gooseberry Cream

Lush, ripe gooseberries capture the essence of the best of British soft summer fruit. Abundant in August, gooseberries are easy to freeze and make lovely sauces, soufflés and pies.

Serves 8

ELDERFLOWER CREAM
11.7g/¹/₂oz sachet (US 1 tablespoon) of powdered
   gelatine dissolved in 60ml/2fl oz/¹/₄ cup of boiling
   water, or vegetarian equivalent
100ml/3¹/₂fl oz/scant ¹/₂ cup of elderflower and lemon
   cordial
550g/1lb 3oz/4 cups of trimmed, ripe dessert
   gooseberries

2 tablespoons of caster (superfine) sugar
2 large free-range eggs, separated
200ml/7fl oz/³/₄ cup of coconut cream
240ml/8fl oz/1 cup of soya cream

Fresh mint leaves and sifted icing (confectioners')
   sugar to decorate

Mix the dissolved gelatine with the elderflower cordial.

Cook the gooseberries with the sugar and a tiny amount of water, just enough so that the fruit will not stick to the pan. When the fruit is bursting and soft, remove from the heat.

When the fruit is nearly cold, place in the food processor and beat to a thick purée. Sieve the purée into a bowl in order to remove all the pips.

Stir the egg yolks and gelatine into the fruit purée and mix thoroughly. Mix in the coconut cream and soya cream.

In another bowl, whisk the egg whites until stiff and then fold into the purée using a metal spoon.

Fill a large pretty bowl or dish with the elderflower and gooseberry cream and leave it to chill in the freezer for about 30–40 minutes.

Once it is starting to set, cover the dish with clingfilm (plastic wrap) and chill it for at least 4 more hours in the refrigerator.

Once the elderflower cream is completely set, decorate it with little sprigs of fresh mint.

At the last moment, dust the elderflower and gooseberry cream with sifted icing (confectioners') sugar. Serve chilled with some crunchy (GF & DF) cookies.

Chocolate and Chestnut Pavé

This is ideal for Christmas or New Year entertaining as it is intensely rich, easy to prepare and can be made a day in advance, which is always useful when the house is full of demanding guests.

Serves 10

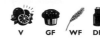

425g/15oz can of unsweetened chestnut purée
200ml/7fl oz/³/₄ cup of golden syrup (corn syrup)
310g/11oz of (DF/GF) continental dark chocolate,
   finely chopped in a food processor
55g/2oz/¹/₄ cup of (DF) margarine, sliced up

225g/8oz/1 ¹/₃ cups of peeled and chopped chestnuts

A loaf/terrine tin lined with clingfilm (plastic wrap)
Sieved (DF/GF) cocoa powder and fresh physalis fruits
   (Cape gooseberries) to decorate

Gently heat the chestnut purée in a non-stick saucepan with the syrup, stirring until smooth and well blended. Add the chopped chocolate and stir until melted and thoroughly mixed.
Remove from the heat and stir in the margarine until it has melted and blended in. Mix in the chestnuts and cool slightly. Spoon the mixture into the prepared loaf or terrine tin.
When the mixture is cold, cover it with foil and chill for 1 hour in the freezer, then another hour in the refrigerator. Leave it in the refrigerator until you are ready to serve it.
Turn out the pavé and peel off the clingfilm (plastic wrap). Serve one slice per person on each plate and decorate with sifted cocoa powder and a couple of physalis (Cape gooseberries) with the wings peeled back for effect.

Chocolate Sorbet

A blissfully sinful sorbet, not remotely slimming, but quite delicious with cookies or Almond Petit Fours (see page 190).

Serves 6

200g/7oz/1 cup of caster (superfine) sugar
140g/5oz of (DF/GF) continental dark chocolate
A pinch of salt
1 teaspoon of ground cinnamon
600ml/20fl oz/2½ cups of water
1 tablespoon of rum

90ml/3fl oz/⅓ cup of fresh strong black coffee
100g/3½ oz/¾ cup of plump raisins

Fresh sprigs of rosemary and seasonal berries or
fruits for decoration

Simmer all the ingredients – except the rum, coffee and the raisins – in a heavy-bottomed pan and bring to the boil. Continue to cook for 5 minutes and then strain into a bowl.

Add the rum, coffee and raisins, and allow to cool.

Churn and freeze the sorbet in an ice-cream maker for 20 minutes, or until frozen but manageable.

Scrape into a sealable container and freeze until needed.

Serve the sorbet straight from the freezer.

A couple of scoops on a plate with some fresh rosemary leaves and a little display of seasonal fresh fruit looks great.

Brandy Snap Baskets

These baskets are brilliant for summer dinner parties – fill with a scoop of Stem Ginger Ice-cream (see page 177) and top with fresh raspberries and a sprig of fresh mint to decorate.

Serves 6

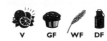

Oil for greasing
55g/2oz/¼ cup of (DF) margarine
55g/2oz/scant ¼ cup of caster (superfine) sugar
2 tablespoons of golden syrup (corn syrup)
55g/2oz/scant ½ cup of white rice flour
1 teaspoon of ground ginger

1 teaspoon of brandy or lemon juice
The grated rind of ½ a lemon

2–3 baking sheets, lined with baking parchment (wax paper)

Preheat the oven to 180°C/350°F/Gas mark 4

Grease the outsides of 6 upturned ramekins.
Melt the margarine with the sugar and the syrup in a small saucepan over a low heat. Remove from the heat and stir in the flour and ginger, brandy or lemon juice and lemon rind.
Place small spoonfuls about 5cm/2 inches apart on the baking sheets to allow for spreading during baking. Cook until golden and bubbly.
Cool for 30 seconds and then speedily loosen them with a greased palette knife and wrap around the ramekin bases.
Leave to set and then carefully prise them off. If they are too brittle then briefly re-heat in the oven and try again.
They are now ready to serve or store in an airtight container.

Double Chocolate Chip Ice-cream

Totally sinful ice-cream! For extra calories serve with cookies or Chocolate Brownies (see page 198).

Serves 4

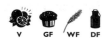

4 large free-range egg yolks
1 heaped teaspoon of (GF) cornflour (cornstarch)
1 heaped tablespoon of sugar
300ml/10fl oz/1¼ cups of soya milk

3 tablespoons of (DF/GF) cocoa powder, sieved
240ml/8fl oz/1 cup of soya cream
100g/3½oz/⅔ cup of (DF/GF) dark chocolate chips or chopped pieces

Mix the egg yolks, cornflour (cornstarch) and sugar together in a bowl. Gradually add the milk. Now transfer this mixture into a non-stick saucepan and cook over a low heat, stirring most of the time until thick – but do not boil.

Remove the pan from the heat and stir in the cocoa powder and soya cream. Sieve the custard into a bowl and leave to cool.

When it is cold and the ice-cream maker is ready, mix in the chocolate chips or pieces and churn in the machine until frozen, but still soft enough to scrape out of the mixer. Freeze in a sealable container until needed, or serve immediately with cookies.

Stem Ginger Ice-cream

For a glamorous pudding, serve with Brandy Snap Baskets (see page 175), or Stem Ginger Cookies (see page 187) and decorate with fresh fruit and mint leaves.

Serves 4

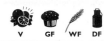

V	GF	WF	DF

1 teaspoon of ground ginger

4 large free-range egg yolks

1 heaped teaspoon of (GF) cornflour (cornstarch)

1 heaped tablespoon of sugar

300ml/10fl oz/1 ¼ cups of soya milk

6 stem ginger, finely chopped

3 tablespoons of stem ginger syrup

240ml/8fl oz/1 cup of soya cream

Mix the ground ginger, egg yolks, cornflour (cornstarch) and sugar together in a bowl and gradually incorporate the milk. Transfer to a non-stick saucepan and, stirring all the time, cook over a low heat until thick and creamy – but do not boil.

Remove from the heat and add the stem ginger, syrup and lastly the soya cream.

Following the instructions on your ice-cream maker, churn until the custard is frozen and serve.

Coconut Ice-cream

To make this a tropical concoction serve with an exotic fruit purée, such as mango, lime juice and passion fruit liquidized together with a little rum, instead of the chocolate sauce.

Serves 6

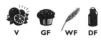

CHOCOLATE SAUCE
140g/5oz of (DF/GF) dark chocolate
100ml/3fl oz/⅓ cup of weak black coffee
140ml/5fl oz/⅔ cup of warm water
2 tablespoons of Amaretto di Saronno liqueur
3 heaped tablespoons of (DF/GF) cocoa powder
2 heaped teaspoons of caster (superfine) sugar

ICE-CREAM
4 large free-range egg yolks
1 heaped teaspoon of (GF) cornflour (cornstarch)
2 heaped tablespoons of caster (superfine) sugar
400ml/14fl oz/1½ cups of coconut milk
5 heaped tablespoons of desiccated (shredded) coconut
200ml/7fl oz/¾ cup of coconut cream
2 tablespoons of toasted coconut pieces (from health food shops)

Make the chocolate sauce by slowly melting together all the sauce ingredients in a non-stick saucepan. Stir until thick and creamy. Remove from the heat and cover until needed.

Make the ice-cream by mixing the egg yolks, cornflour (cornstarch) and sugar together in a bowl, and slowly adding the coconut milk. Transfer to a saucepan, add the desiccated (shredded) coconut and cook over a low heat, stirring all the time. Cook until thick and smooth, then remove from the heat and transfer to a bowl. Stir in the coconut cream.

Once it is cool, pour the custard into your prepared ice-cream maker and churn until frozen and smooth (probably about 20 minutes).

Serve scoops of ice-cream scattered with toasted coconut pieces with a pool of lukewarm chocolate sauce beside it.

Lemon Curd Ice-cream

This is such a refreshing ice-cream that I often make large quantities. It is perfect for bigger parties outside in the garden in the summer or barbecues for teenagers.

Serves about 16

LEMON CURD

Zest and juice from 4 unwaxed lemons

4 large free-range eggs and 4 large free-range egg yolks

300g/10½oz/1½ cups of caster (superfine) sugar

200g/7oz/1 cup of (DF) margarine

ICE-CREAM

100g/3½oz/1 cup of chopped citrus peel soaked in 2 tablespoons of Cointreau for up to 24 hours before use

4 or 5 x 227g/8oz tubs of thick sheep's yogurt

All the lemon curd

2 large free-range egg whites

Make the lemon curd first (this can be made up to a week in advance and kept sealed in the refrigerator). Beat the lemon zest and juice with the eggs, egg yolks and sugar in a non-stick saucepan. Place on medium heat and stir the mixture until it warms up and the sugar dissolves. Bring the mixture to boiling point but do not boil, it should be very thick. Remove from the heat immediately, add all the margarine and stir vigorously until it is thoroughly incorporated.

Stir frequently while the lemon curd cools down. Transfer to a sealable container and chill until needed. The curd must be cold before it is added to the ice-cream.

Marinate the citrus peel in a little bowl, the day before if possible. Keep it cool and covered until needed.

Make sure your ice-cream maker is ready when you want to make the ice-cream. If you like a strong lemon flavour then use the smaller amount of yogurt and if you prefer it a little less zingy then use the 5 tubs.

Whisk the yogurt with the lemon curd in a very large mixing bowl for at least 6 minutes at medium speed. It will become lighter and slightly increased in volume.

Whisk the egg whites until very stiff and then fold into the curd mixture. Fold in the citrus peel and Cointreau.

Churn the ice-cream in 2 batches until frozen. Transfer to a sealable container and freeze until needed.

You can either buy little (GF) meringue nests to serve the ice-cream in for dinner parties or you can serve it in (GF) Brandy Snap Baskets (*see page 175*).

Praline Ice-cream

This is the ice-cream I miss most as I always see it in the supermarkets. It is ideal with any fruit or for dinner parties scooped into meringue baskets or Brandy Snap Baskets (see page 175).

Serves 6

55g/2oz/scant ¼ cup of caster (superfine) sugar
55g/2oz/½ cup of chopped blanched almonds
1 teaspoon (GF) cornflour (cornstarch)
4 large free-range egg yolks

300ml/10fl oz/1¼ cups of soya milk
1 vanilla pod, split
240ml/8fl oz/1 cup of soya cream
1 teaspoon of pure Madagascan vanilla extract

Make the praline first by quickly melting the sugar with the almonds in a saucepan until they turn dark golden brown. Leave the mixture to cool. When the praline is cold put it into a plastic bag and bash with a rolling pin until it resembles breadcrumbs (alternatively grind to a powder in a food processor).

Now make the ice-cream by quickly mixing the cornflour (cornstarch) with the egg yolks and a little of the milk until you have a smooth paste. Continue adding the milk and then pour the liquid into a saucepan to cook. Add the vanilla pod and then stir continuously until the custard is very thick and hot – but do not boil.

Remove the pan from the heat and take out the pod (wash it under warm water, then dry it so that you can re-use it).

Now add the cream and blend briefly. Mix in the vanilla extract and the praline and leave to cool.

Follow the instructions on your ice-cream maker and pour in the custard. Churn until frozen and then serve, or freeze in a sealable container.

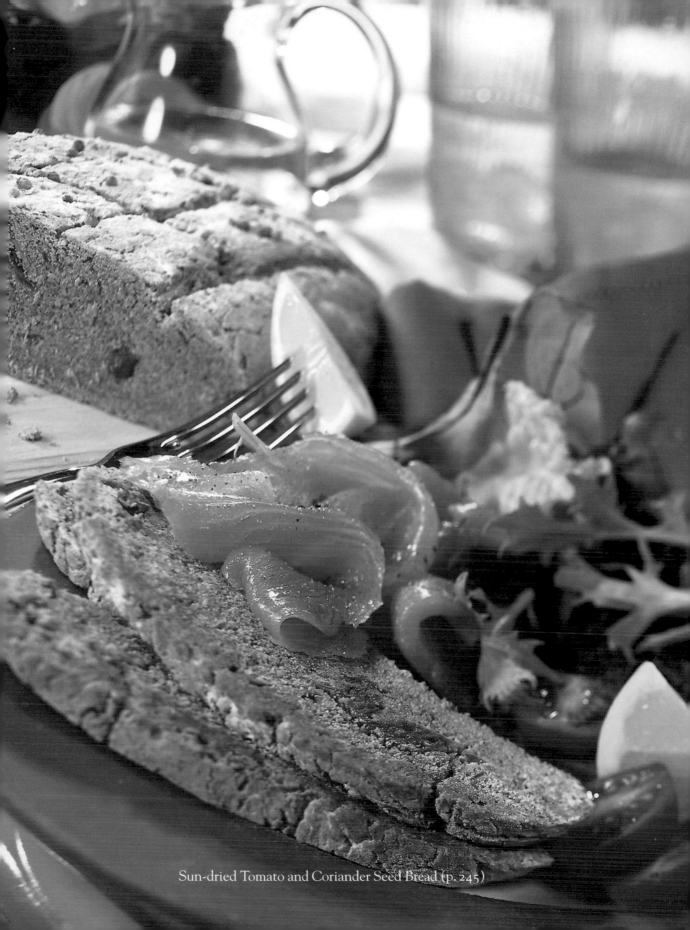

Sun-dried Tomato and Coriander Seed Bread (p. 245)

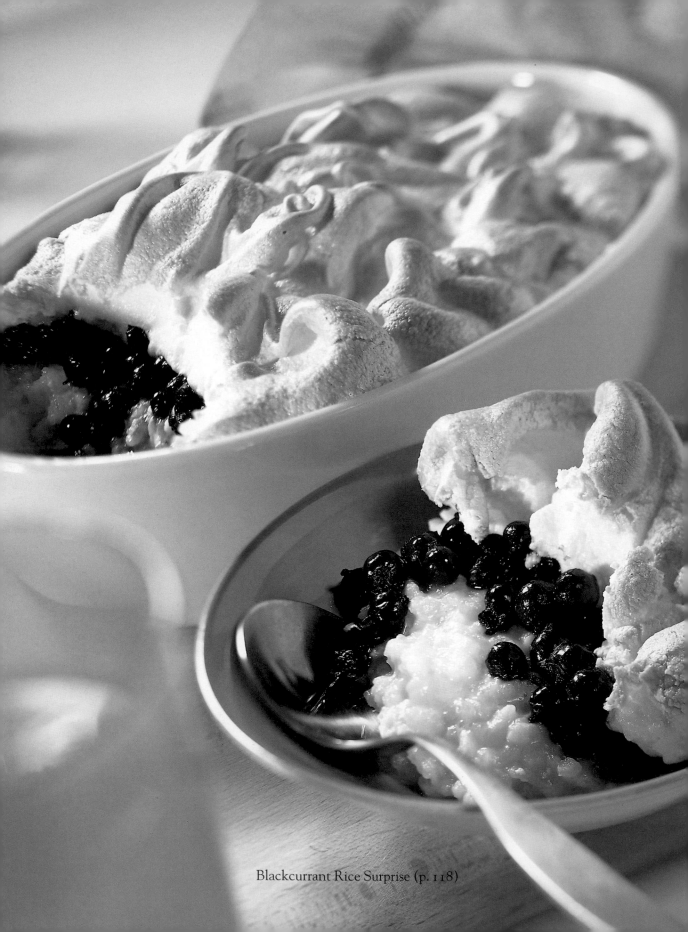

Blackcurrant Rice Surprise (p. 118)

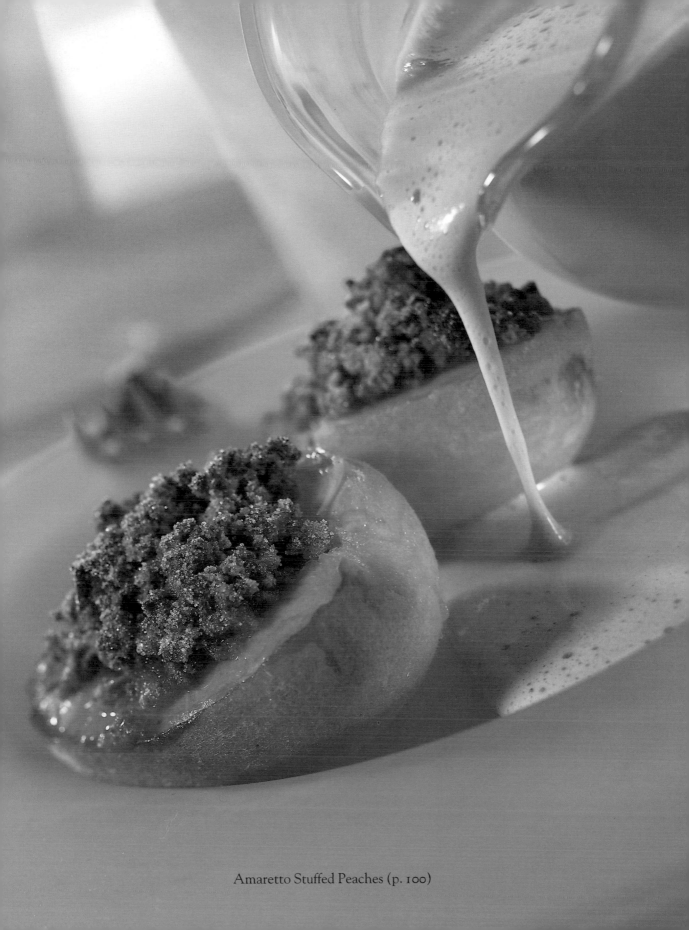

Amaretto Stuffed Peaches (p. 100)

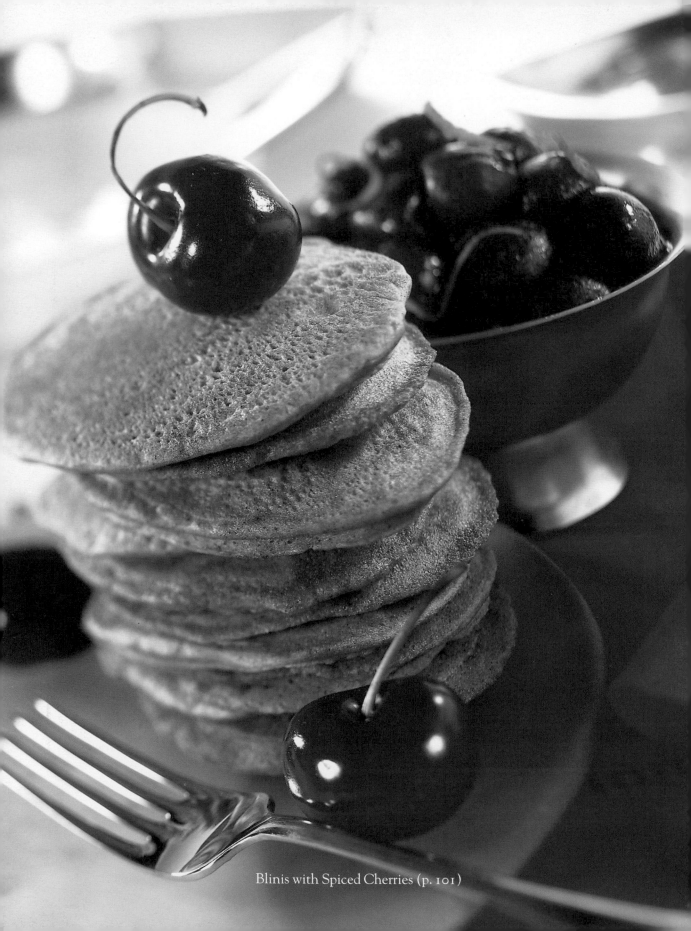

Blinis with Spiced Cherries (p. 101)

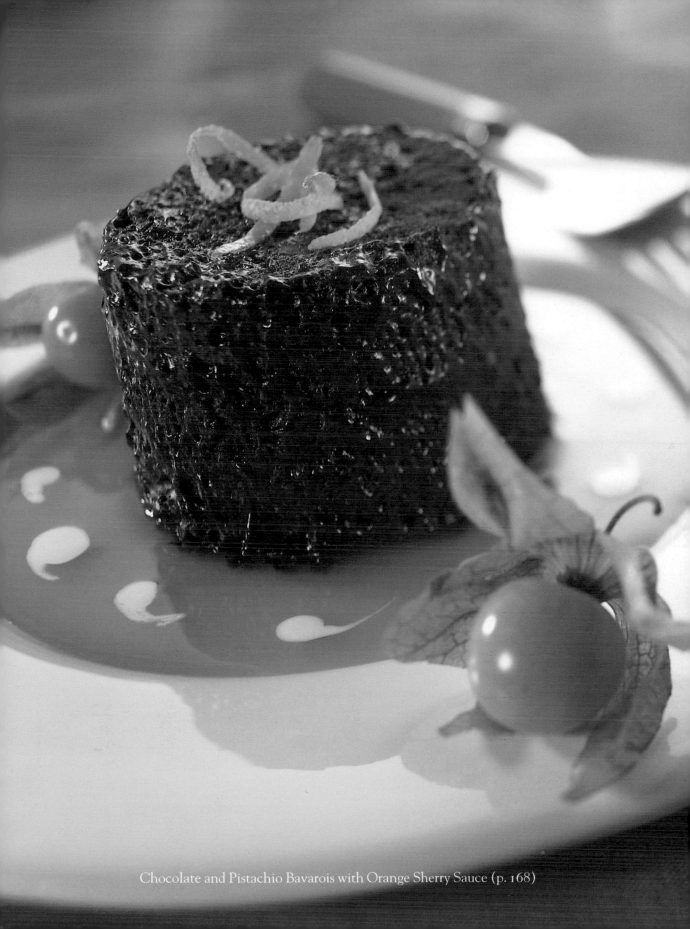

Chocolate and Pistachio Bavarois with Orange Sherry Sauce (p. 168)

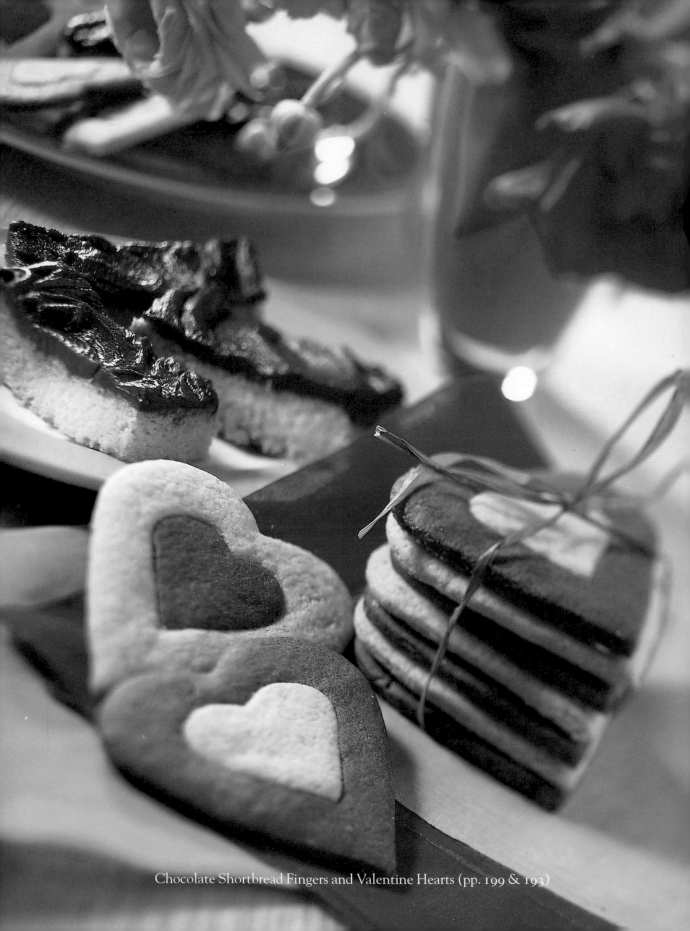

Chocolate Shortbread Fingers and Valentine Hearts (pp. 199 & 193)

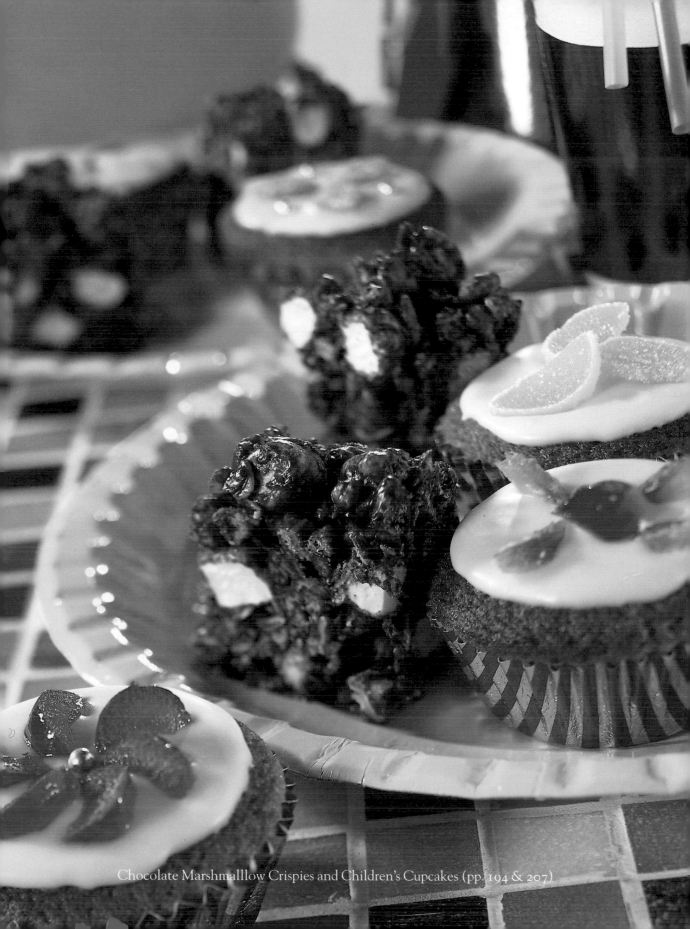

Chocolate Marshmalllow Crispies and Children's Cupcakes (pp.194 & 207)

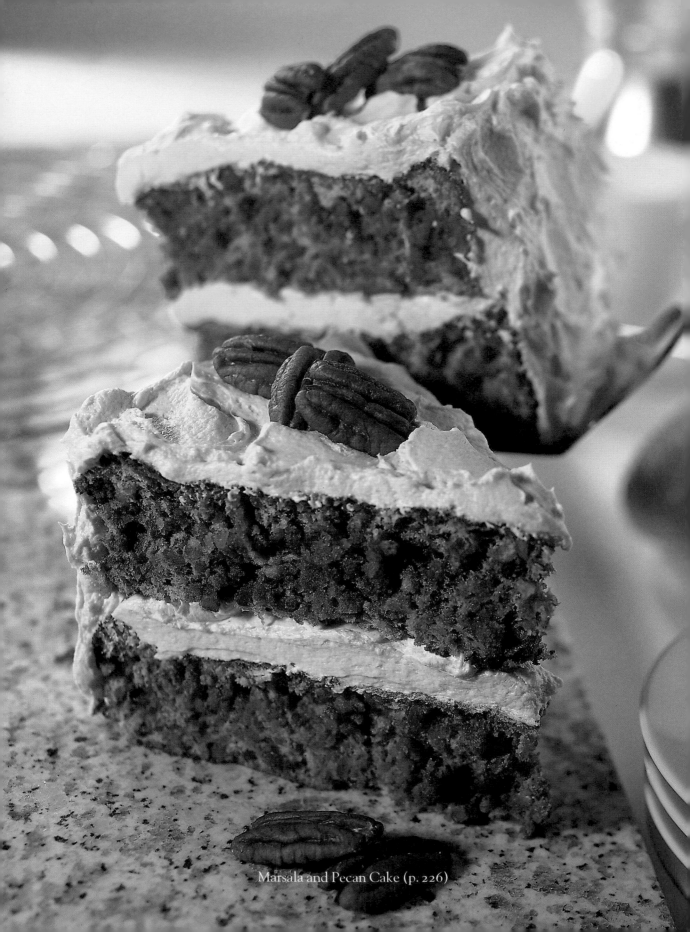

Marsala and Pecan Cake (p. 226)

Banana and Pecan Ice-cream with Damson Coulis

Autumn starts when the damsons appear, heralding the rich colours of the season. This luscious purple fruit is a dramatic contrast to the pale ice-cream it is served with. A variation of this dish can be made at any time of year by using the out-of-season sauce.

Serves 8–12

V   GF   WF   DF

DAMSON COULIS

500g/17oz/4 cups of damsons, stalks and any bad
   patches removed
4 or more tablespoons of caster (superfine) sugar
   (increase to suit taste)
4 tablespoons of damson gin, sloe gin or white rum
Water and more of the chosen spirit to correct the
   consistency if necessary

QUICK OUT-OF-SEASON SAUCE

450g/16oz jar of forest fruits or stoned (pitted)
   black cherries in liqueur or brandy
or
450g/16oz can of soft red fruits or black cherries
   in natural juices

ICE-CREAM

5 large free-range egg yolks
2 teaspoons of (GF) cornflour (cornstarch)
2 tablespoons of caster (superfine) sugar
500ml/17fl oz/2 cups of soya cream
2 teaspoons of (GF) mixed (pie) spice
100g/3½oz/¾ cup of chopped pecan nuts
4 tablespoons of pure maple syrup
2 tablespoons of brandy
4 large, ripe, mashed bananas in the juice of
   ½ a lemon

Make the damson coulis by gently cooking the fruit, sugar and gin in a pan, over medium heat, until the fruit is soft. Add water if the damsons start to stick, but only add a little at a time, otherwise the sauce will be too runny.

Let the fruit get cold, then pass the fruit and its liquid through a sieve into a bowl. Discard the fruit skins and stones. Add more sugar, water or additional alcohol to taste, and to achieve the perfect consistency.

Transfer the coulis to a serving jug and chill until needed.

If damsons are unavailable, use the fruits suggested for the out-of-season sauce and liquidize them in their juices.

Sieve the sauce to remove any pips or skins, place in a serving jug and chill until needed.

To make the ice-cream, beat the egg yolks with the cornflour (cornstarch) and sugar in a non-stick saucepan. Gradually incorporate the soya cream, mixed (pie) spice and pecans.

Stir the custard over low heat until it comes to the boil, then remove from the heat and stir in the maple syrup and brandy.

Let the mixture cool slightly and then stir in the mashed bananas and lemon juice.

Once the mixture is cool, and your ice-cream maker is ready, churn the ice-cream for about 20 minutes or until it is frozen.

Scrape out the ice-cream and store in an airtight container in the freezer until needed.

Serve the ice-cream in a large scoop with the damson or fruit coulis poured all around it.

Christmas Pudding Ice-cream

Here is an ideal way of using up Christmas pudding leftovers and getting away with serving it as a party piece! Decorate it as ostentatiously as you like to suit the occasion.

Serves 6

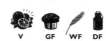

V GF WF DF

6 heaped tablespoons of leftover (GF&DF) Christmas pudding

8 small free-range egg yolks

1 tablespoon of (GF) cornflour (cornstarch)

2 heaped tablespoons of caster (superfine) sugar

1 teaspoon of pure Madagascan vanilla extract

300ml/10fl oz/1¼ cups of soya milk

225ml/7½ fl oz/generous ¾ cup of soya cream

200ml/7fl oz/¾ cup of coconut cream

3 tablespoons of rum

Clingfilm (plastic wrap)

A sprig of holly for decoration

Line a pudding basin with clingfilm (plastic wrap). Crumble up the leftover Christmas pudding and put it into a large bowl. Mix the eggs in a separate bowl with the cornflour (cornstarch), sugar and vanilla extract. Gradually add the milk until it is all well blended. Transfer the mixture to a non-stick saucepan and cook slowly, stirring often, until it becomes very thick.

Let the custard come to the boil, remove it from the heat and stir in the soya cream, coconut cream and the rum. Pass the custard through a fine sieve into the bowl of Christmas pudding. Gently mix it all together, then allow the mixture to cool.

When the ice-cream maker is ready, churn the custard and Christmas pudding mixture until frozen but still soft enough to scrape out of the bowl.

Spoon the ice-cream into the lined basin, smooth over and seal with the clingfilm (plastic wrap). Freeze for 4 hours or more.

Remove the clingfilm (plastic wrap) from the pudding and turn out onto a plate. Peel off the remaining clingfilm (plastic wrap), put a sprig of holly on top and serve immediately.

CHAPTER 10

Cookies, Cakes and Sweets

Chocolate Chip and Brazil Nut Cookies

Brilliant bribery for children of all ages! You can vary the chocolate chips if you can eat milk and white chocolate and you can vary the nuts to peanuts, hazelnuts, pecans or walnuts. For a nut-free version, use chopped dried apricots or other fruit or berries with seeds.

Makes 16–20

V   GF   WF   DF

125g/4¹/₂oz/generous ³/₄ cup of *Wellfoods* (WF) flour
¹/₂ teaspoon of bicarbonate of soda (baking soda)
55g/2oz/¹/₄ cup of soft brown sugar
55g/2oz/¹/₄ cup of vanilla sugar (or add 1 teaspoon of vanilla extract to ordinary sugar)
70g/2¹/₂oz/¹/₃ cup of (DF) margarine

1 large free-range egg
55g/2oz/¹/₃ cup of chopped Brazil nuts
100g/3¹/₂oz of (DF/GF) dark chocolate, chopped into small pieces

3 greased baking sheets

Preheat the oven to 180°C/350°F/Gas mark 4

Combine the first 6 ingredients in a food processor and blend for a few seconds. Mix in the nuts and chocolate.
Spoon small mounds of the mixture onto the greased baking sheets and keep them well spaced out. Bake the cookies for 7–10 minutes until golden brown. Leave for 2 minutes then lift them off and place them on a wire rack to cool.

Stem Ginger Cookies

Grown-up ginger cookies that have a habit of disappearing before they even get to the cookie jar!

 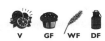

100g/3½oz/7 tablespoons of (DF) margarine
100g/3½oz/½ cup of caster (superfine) sugar
3 tablespoons of black treacle (molasses)
3 tablespoons of golden syrup (corn syrup)
1 large free-range egg, beaten
70g/2½oz/½ cup of rice flour
200g/7oz/scant 1½ cups of buckwheat flour
2 teaspoons of bicarbonate of soda (baking soda)

2 teaspoons each of ground ginger and
   ground cinnamon
¼ teaspoon of salt
5 tablespoons of water
5 pieces of stem ginger, finely chopped

3 greased baking sheets

Preheat the oven to 200°C/400°F/Gas mark 6

Cream the margarine and sugar together until light and fluffy. Beat in the treacle (molasses), syrup, egg and remaining ingredients.

Drop half tablespoons of the mixture 5cm/2 inches apart on the baking sheets and bake for 6–8 minutes.

Remove the cookies from the sheets and allow to cool on a wire rack.

Peanut Butter Cookies

You can add chunks of (DF/GF) dark chocolate to vary these cookies. I find them remarkably efficient as bribery when my God-children come to stay!

Makes 24

100g/3¹/₂oz/²/₃ cup of rice flour
130g/4¹/₂oz/generous ³/₄ cup of maize flour
¹/₂ teaspoon of salt
¹/₂ teaspoon of bicarbonate of soda (baking soda)
100g/3¹/₂oz/7 tablespoons of (DF) margarine
130g/4¹/₂oz/¹/₂ cup of (GF/DF) crunchy peanut butter

170g/6oz/³/₄ cup of soft brown sugar
2 large free-range eggs
1 teaspoon of pure Madagascan vanilla extract
1 teaspoon of water
100g/3¹/₂oz/¹/₂ cup of dry-roasted peanuts

Preheat oven to 180°C/350°F/Gas mark 4

Sift the flours with the salt and bicarbonate of soda (baking soda) onto a plate and set aside. In a large bowl, cream the margarine, peanut butter and sugar until soft and light. Gently mix in half the eggs, the vanilla extract and water, and then stir in half the flour. Repeat so that they are all used up, then add the peanuts.

Drop heaped spoonfuls of the dough on to non-stick baking trays and press with the back of a floured fork to flatten slightly.

Bake them for 15 minutes. Allow the cookies to cool a little on the tray, before transferring them to a wire rack to cool completely.

Banana and Chocolate Chip Cookies

This is such a good way of using up brown, overripe bananas that no one else in the house will eat.

Makes 24

170g/6oz/1¼ cups of rice flour

170g/6oz/1¼ cups of oat flour (or finely processed oats)

1 heaped teaspoon of bicarbonate of soda (baking soda)

A pinch of salt

255g/9oz/1 cup plus 2 tablespoons of (DF) margarine, diced

140g/5oz/¾ cup of demerara sugar

100g/3½oz/½ cup of granulated sugar

2 large free-range eggs

1 teaspoon of pure Madagascan vanilla extract

2 small ripe bananas, mashed

85g/3oz/¾ cup of banana chips, roughly broken up

115g/4oz/⅔ cup of (DF/GF) dark chocolate drops or chopped pieces

Preheat the oven to 190°C/375°F/Gas mark 5

Sift the flours, bicarbonate of soda (baking soda) and salt into a bowl and set aside.
In a food processor, beat the margarine and both the sugars until light and fluffy. Gradually add the eggs, followed by the vanilla extract. Transfer the mixture to a large bowl, stir in the mashed bananas and fold in the flour as lightly as you can. Fold in the banana chips and chocolate pieces. Drop tablespoons of the mixture on to a non-stick baking tray, spacing the cookies well apart. Bake them for 15 minutes, or until golden brown.
Cool the cookies slightly before lifting them onto a wire rack. When they are cold, store in an airtight container until needed.

Almond Petit Fours

Here are perfect little petit fours to nibble with coffee or to accompany ice-cream or sorbet as a pudding. They are also good finely crushed and mixed into meringue or vanilla ice-cream. You can freeze them or keep them for up to a week in a sealable container.

Serves about 20

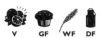

225g/8oz/1 ½ cups of whole skinned almonds
255g/9oz/1 ¼ cups of caster (superfine) sugar
½ a finely grated orange
2 medium free-range egg whites
20 large glacé cherries, halved

Icing (confectioners') sugar to dust
Sheets of rice paper

Preheat the oven to 180°C/350°F/Gas mark 4

Put the almonds in a food processor and grind briefly. Add half the caster (superfine) sugar and grind again until it becomes a powder. Mix with the remaining caster (superfine) sugar and the grated orange zest. Transfer the mixture to a bowl.

In another bowl, whisk the egg whites lightly with an electric whisk, then stir the egg whites into the almond mixture to bind it.

Take heaped teaspoons of the mixture and roll it into balls, on a board dusted with icing (confectioners') sugar.

Flatten the balls with a palette knife and press half a cherry into the centre of each. Place them well apart on a baking sheet lined with rice paper.

Bake for 15 minutes or until just firm but pale golden brown.

Cool on the baking sheets and then trim the rice paper around the biscuits. Serve the petit fours on the day of baking, dusted with icing (confectioners') sugar.

Chocolate Macaroons

These are the perfect accompaniment to lots of different types of ice-cream. The macaroons are quick to make so they are also an ideal foundation for trifles and mousse-cakes.

Makes 24

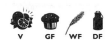

200g/7oz/1 ⅓ cups of whole almonds
55g/2oz of (DF/GF) plain chocolate
130g/4½oz/½ cups plus 2 tablespoons of caster
   (superfine) sugar
1 teaspoon of pure Madagascan vanilla extract
½ teaspoon of almond essence

1 tablespoon of (DF/GF) cocoa powder
2 large free-range egg whites

Icing (confectioners') sugar for dusting your hands
   and the board
Sheets of rice paper

Preheat the oven to 180°C/350°F/Gas mark 4

Bake the almonds for a few minutes until pale gold. Allow them to cool. Gently melt the chocolate in a bowl in the microwave.

Grind the cooled nuts in a food processor to a fine powder. Add the caster (superfine) sugar, vanilla extract, almond essence, cocoa powder, melted chocolate and egg whites and mix to a soft paste.

Put plenty of icing (confectioners') sugar on a clean board and roll the mixture into a long sausage. With plenty of icing (confectioners') sugar on your hands, shape slices of the dough into balls the size of walnuts.

Arrange the macaroons on sheets of rice paper on some non-stick baking trays and bake for 15 minutes, or until just firm.

Cool the cookies slightly and then cut the rice paper around the cookies and cool them on a wire rack. These macaroons are best eaten on the day of baking.

Orange Maple Cookies

These richly flavoured Canadian-style cookies use maple syrup, but for a cheaper version substitute honey.

Serves 12

100g/3½oz/⅔ cup of rice flour
100g/3½oz/⅔ cup of maize flour
100g/3½oz/⅔ cup of millet flour
115g/4oz/½ cup (DF) margarine, softened
70g/2½oz/⅓ cup of unrefined dark Mauritian sugar
4 tablespoons of pure maple syrup
1 teaspoon of (GF) cream of tartar

½ teaspoon of (GF) bicarbonate of soda (baking soda)
1 large free-range egg
1 tablespoon of grated orange rind

2 non-stick baking trays, greased and floured

Preheat the oven to 180°C/350°F/Gas mark 4

In a large bowl, mix all the ingredients with an electric whisk. When the mixture has formed a dough, shape into a ball with your hands, then wrap in clingfilm (plastic wrap) and refrigerate for 1 hour.

Roll out the dough, half at a time, until about 3mm/⅛-inch thick. Cut into the required shapes and place 2.5cm/1 inch apart on the trays. Bake the cookies for 10 minutes, or until they are golden.

Transfer on to wire racks to cool. Store the cookies in an airtight container until needed.

Valentine Hearts

These eye-catching little hearts make a fun gift, or amusing cookies to serve with ice-cream or mousses on St. Valentine's day.

Makes 2¹/2 – 3¹/2 dozen

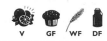

100g/3¹/2oz of (DF/GF) dark chocolate	2 non-stick baking sheets
170g/6oz/1¹/4 cups of rice flour	2 heart-shaped cutters, one 5cm/2 inch and the other
170g/6oz/1¹/4 cups of millet flour	2.5cm/1 inch (fluted circular cutters can be used
170g/6oz/³/4 cup of (DF) margarine	instead)
1 tablespoon of strong black coffee	
2 teaspoons of (GF) baking powder	
1 large free-range egg	
140g/5oz/³/4 cup of caster (superfine) sugar	

Preheat the oven to 180°C/350°F/Gas mark 4

Gently melt the chocolate in a bowl in the microwave and then stir it until smooth.

In a food processor, combine the flours and margarine with the coffee for a few seconds. Add the baking powder, egg and sugar, and process again briefly.

Shape the dough into a ball, divide into two and wrap one in clingfilm (plastic wrap). Chill the wrapped dough for 25 minutes in the freezer.

Mix the melted chocolate into the remaining dough and bring it back into a ball shape by kneading gently on a floured surface. Wrap the chocolate dough in clingfilm (plastic wrap) and freeze for 15 minutes.

Unwrap both balls of dough and divide each in half to make it easier to roll out.

Now roll out a chocolate dough and a plain dough on separate, floured boards until they are thin enough to cut out without breaking up.

Using the large heart cutter first, cut out plenty of hearts in the chocolate pastry, then using the smaller heart cutter, cut out the centre of the chocolate hearts and put them to one side.

Repeat this with the plain dough. Now gently place the smaller hearts inside the larger ones, alternating doughs so that you have a chocolate exterior and a plain interior and a plain exterior and a chocolate interior.

Bake the hearts on the trays for about 10 minutes, or until golden. Allow them to cool for a couple of minutes before transferring to wire racks.

Chocolate Marshmallow Crispies

Children on school holidays with time on their hands and a sense of creativity can try making these simple cookies for tea.

Makes 12

170g/6oz/³/₄ cup of (DF) margarine

140g/5oz of (DF/GF) chocolate

85g/3oz/¹/₄ cup of golden syrup (corn syrup)

140g/5oz/4¹/₂ cups of (WF) Rice Crispies
   (puffed rice cereal)

170g/6oz/1¹/₂ cups of rolled oats

100g/3¹/₂oz/2 cups of chopped or mini
   marshmallows

Place the margarine, chocolate and syrup in a non-stick saucepan and heat gently until melted and blended together.

Cool the mixture before adding the rice crispies, oats and marshmallows.

Mix well and then press the crispies into 12 paper baking cups or a 20cm/8 inch square non-stick baking tin.

Chill for 30 minutes and mark out portions in the tin. Chill for at least 2 hours in the freezer before serving. Keep the crispies cool otherwise there will be lots of very sticky fingers!

Nutmeg Cookies

You can use any spice you like for these little cookies – simply change it according to the type of fruits, mousses or ices you are serving.

Makes 30

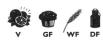

200g/7oz/1 cup less 2 tablespoons of (DF)
  margarine
85g/3oz/generous 1/2 cup of icing (confectioners')
  sugar
100g/3 1/2oz/2/3 cup of rice flour
100g/3 1/2oz/2/3 cup of (GF) cornflour (cornstarch)
55g/2oz/2/3 cup of ground almonds

1 teaspoon of finely grated nutmeg
Finely grated zest of 1/2 a lemon

2 baking trays, lined with baking parchment
  (wax paper)
Extra flour for dusting hands and board

Preheat the oven to 180°C/350°F/Gas mark 4

Cream the margarine and icing (confectioners') sugar in a food processor, then add all the remaining ingredients, giving them a quick blend until a dough forms.
With floured hands, wrap the ball of dough in clingfilm (plastic wrap) and chill for 2 hours.
Roll the dough into a long sausage shape on a floured board and cut it into 30 slices. Place the slices on the prepared tray, making sure that the cookies have room to expand.
Bake the cookies for about 15 minutes, or until lightly coloured around the edges.
Cool the cookies slightly, then transfer them to a wire tray to cool.
Store the cookies in an airtight container until needed.

Coconut Crunches

These are wonderful with sorbets, or just with afternoon tea or coffee.

Serves 6–10

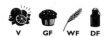

140g/5oz/1²/₃ cups of desiccated (shredded) coconut
3 egg whites
3 tablespoons of caster (superfine) sugar

1 tablespoon of (GF) cornflour (cornstarch)
1 teaspoon of orange flower water

Set the oven at 180°C/350°F/Gas mark 4

Mix all of the ingredients together to form a firm paste.
Using a spoon and your fingers, shape the dough into walnut size balls and place them on a non-stick baking sheet. Bake in the middle of the oven for 10 minutes and then reduce the heat to 150°C/300°F/Gas mark 2 and bake for a further 5 minutes.
Cool on a wire rack and store in an airtight container until needed.

Gingerbread Men

These traditional cookies can be made into wonderful ornamental decorations at Christmas. Children love to pipe icing on to the gingerbread men.

Makes 20

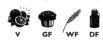

100ml/3½ fl oz/⅓ cup of black treacle (molasses)

55g/2oz/¼ cup of (DF) margarine

55g/2oz/scant ¼ cup of unrefined dark Mauritian sugar

1 teaspoon of bicarbonate of soda (baking soda)

½ teaspoon of allspice

½ teaspoon of ground cinnamon

½ teaspoon of ground cloves

1 teaspoon of ground ginger

1 large free-range egg

130g/4½oz/generous ¾ cup of rice flour

100g/3½oz/⅔ cup of millet flour

100g/3½oz/⅔ cup of potato flour

Icing if used – (GF) ready-to-pipe varieties, silver balls or other (GF/DF) decorations

Preheat the oven to 180°C/350°F/Gas mark 4

In a large bowl, combine the treacle (molasses) and margarine, then melt them together in the microwave. Allow the mixture to cool down, then add the sugar, bicarbonate of soda (baking soda), spices, egg and all the flours.

Beat with a wooden spoon for 2 minutes. Transfer the dough onto a floured board and knead the dough with a little extra flour until you can roll it with a floured rolling pin. Roll out the dough until it is thin enough to cut out the shapes you require. You can use any shape cutters – gingerbread men, Father Christmas, Christmas trees, hearts or stars.

Place the gingerbread men on non-stick baking trays at least 1cm/½ inch apart. Bake for 12 minutes, or until the edges are firm.

Cool on the trays before lifting them off. Transfer the gingerbread men to wire racks to cool completely. Pipe decorative outlines with the icing and decorate with silver balls or anything you fancy, as long as you check that the ingredients are compatible with you. The icing will take about 1 hour to dry.

The gingerbread men will keep for a couple of days if stored in an airtight container.

Chocolate Brownies

My absolute favourite! Chewy brownies with (DF) vanilla ice-cream was my daily fix when I lived in New York.

Serves 6

70g/2¹/₂oz/¹/₃ cup of (DF) margarine

100g/3¹/₂oz of (DF/GF) dark chocolate

170g/6oz/generous ³/₄ cup of caster (superfine) sugar

2 large free-range eggs, beaten

70g/2¹/₂oz/¹/₂ cup of rice flour

1 teaspoon of (GF) baking powder

¹/₄ teaspoon of salt

¹/₂ teaspoon of pure Madagascan vanilla extract

70g/2¹/₂oz/²/₃ cup of chopped pecan nuts

28cm/11 inch rectangular non-stick baking tin, greased with a little sunflower oil

---

Preheat the oven to 180°C/350°F/Gas mark 4

Melt the margarine and chocolate in a saucepan over a very low heat, stirring constantly. Remove from the heat, add the sugar and allow to cool slightly.

Mix in the beaten eggs, then sift in the flour, baking powder and salt and fold in the vanilla extract and the chopped nuts.

Pour the mixture into the baking tin and bake for 30 minutes. Test with an inserted skewer that it is just cooked through (the skewer should come out clean).

Cool in the tin and cut into squares.

Chocolate Shortbread Fingers

If you can eat dairy products then you can use milk chocolate, which most children prefer.

Makes 6–12

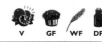

SHORTBREAD
225g/8oz/1 generous cup of caster (superfine) sugar
225g/8oz/2½ cups of ground almonds
225g/8oz/1½ cups of instant quick-cook polenta
   (maize)
225g/8oz/1 cup of (DF) margarine
1 teaspoon of almond essence

CHOCOLATE TOPPING
140g/5oz of (DF/GF) dark chocolate, broken into
   pieces
4 tablespoons of weak black coffee
1 teaspoon of sunflower oil
100g/3½oz/¾ cup of sifted icing (confectioners') sugar

A roulade or Swiss roll non-stick baking tin, lined with
   baking parchment (wax paper)

Preheat the oven to 170°C/325°F/Gas mark 3

Mix all the shortbread ingredients together in a bowl or a food processor until well blended.
Press the mixture evenly into the tin and bake it for 25 minutes until golden and firm to touch.
Cool the shortbread in the tin, then turn it out on to a clean surface and remove the paper.
Melt the chocolate with the coffee in the microwave and stir in the sunflower oil. Beat in the icing (confectioners') sugar and once it is glossy, spread the chocolate over the shortbread.
Make any patterns and squiggles you like to decorate it. Cut the shortbread into fingers or squares and leave it to set in a cool place.
Transfer the shortbread to an airtight container until needed.

Almond Shortbread

This shortbread can be served with any (DF) ice-cream or a bowl of poached fruit, or just with a cup of espresso as a treat!

Serves 6–12

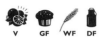

225g/8oz/1 cup of caster (superfine) sugar
225g/8oz/2⅔ cups of ground almonds
225g/8oz/1½ cups of instant quick-cook polenta
225g/8oz/1 cup of (DF) margarine
1 teaspoon of almond essence

2 × 20cm/8 inch loose-bottomed, fluted flan tins

Preheat the oven to 170°C/325°F/Gas mark 3

Mix all of the dry ingredients in a bowl. Mix in the margarine and almond essence until well blended. Press into the tin and spread evenly.
Bake for 25 minutes until golden and firm to the touch. Cool in the tin and then turn out onto a wire rack. Store in an airtight container until needed.

Coffee and Brazil Nut Squares

These cookies are a slight variation of traditional brownies. They freeze well, which is always handy in the school holidays.

Makes 12

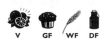

85g/3oz/6 tablespoons of (DF) margarine
200g/7oz/1 cup of demerara sugar
130g/4½oz/generous ¾ cup of rice flour
1½ teaspoons of (GF) baking powder
Pinch of salt
2 large free-range eggs, lightly beaten
1 teaspoon of pure Madagascan vanilla extract
1 heaped teaspoon of instant coffee, dissolved in
   1 tablespoon of boiling water

1 tablespoon of (DF/GF) cocoa powder, dissolved in
   1 tablespoon of boiling water
55g/2oz/½ cup of Brazil nuts, roughly chopped
   and lightly dusted with rice flour
85g/3oz/½ cup of (DF/GF) dark chocolate drops
   or pieces

18 x 25 x 3cm/7 x 10 x 1¼ inch baking tin,
   lightly oiled

Preheat the oven to 190°C/375°F/Gas mark 5

Heat the margarine and sugar together in a pan until it begins to dissolve, then remove from the heat and allow to cool.

Sift the flour, baking powder and salt into a bowl. Mix together the eggs, vanilla extract, coffee and dissolved cocoa in another bowl. Stir the egg mixture into the margarine mixture and then fold in the flour mixture.

Lightly stir in the nuts and chocolate drops or pieces, then pour the mixture into the prepared tin. Bake for 20 minutes, or until the sides are coming away from the edges of the tin. Leave the cake to cool in the tin. When cold, carefully cut the cake into 12 squares and serve, or store in an airtight container until needed.

Coconut and Cinnamon Flapjacks

Perfect flapjacks should keep their shape without crumbling but be gooey enough to have a chewy texture. I alternate taking these to work for a snack with the Coffee and Brazil Nut Squares (see page 201).

Makes 12

200g/7oz/1 cup less 2 tablespoons of (DF) margarine
300g/11oz/scant 1 cup of golden syrup (corn syrup)
400g/14oz/4 cups of porridge oats
85g/3oz/1 cup of desiccated (shredded) coconut
85g/3oz/²/₃ cup of plump sultanas (golden raisins)
1 heaped teaspoon of ground cinnamon

23 x 33cm/9 x 13 inch non-stick Swiss roll or roulade tin, greased and lined with baking parchment (wax paper)

Preheat the oven to 190°C/375°F/Gas mark 5

Melt the margarine with the syrup in a saucepan over medium heat. Add the oats, coconut, sultanas (golden raisins) and cinnamon. Stir the mixture until melted and well blended, then pour it into the roulade tin.

Press the mixture down into the tin, then bake for about 25 minutes, or until golden brown. Cut the flapjacks into squares whilst still warm, but leave them to cool in the tin.

Store the flapjacks in an airtight container until needed.

Sesame Flapjacks

Flapjacks are ideal for picnics because they don't break up easily and they are filling, chewy and healthy. I've included instructions for drizzling with dark chocolate for a naughty snack!

Makes 24

200g/7oz/1 cup less 2 tablespoons of (DF) margarine
300g/10½oz/1 cup of golden syrup (corn syrup)
455g/16oz/5⅓ cups of porridge oats
Pinch of salt
1 heaped tablespoon of sesame seeds

1 tablespoon of finely chopped stem ginger (optional) or 1 heaped teaspoon of ground cinnamon with 100g/3½oz/¾ cup of mincemeat (optional – ideal for Christmas)
140g/5oz of dark (DF/GF) chocolate

Preheat the oven to 180°C/350°F/Gas mark 4

Melt the margarine with the syrup in a saucepan over a low heat, or in the microwave.
Add the oats, salt and sesame seeds, and the stem ginger or the cinnamon and mincemeat if using.
Turn into an oiled baking tin and press down with the back of a spoon.
Bake in the centre of the oven for about 25 minutes, or until golden brown.
Gently heat the chocolate and 2 tablespoons of water together in a bowl over a pan of boiling water. When it is the right consistency, drizzle the mixture over the flapjacks.
Cut into squares whilst hot, but allow to cool completely before removing from the tin to store or serve.

Low-fat Ginger Flapjacks

You can use whichever dried fruits you have in the cupboard, the more exotic the better! Use organic oats – they give a nuttier taste as well as being better for you. If you prefer a subtle ginger flavour, reduce the amount of root and stem (preserved) ginger according to taste.

Serves 6

255g/9oz/2½ cups of organic quick-cooking oats
55g/2oz/scant ¼ cup of brown sugar
5 tablespoons of skimmed milk powder
A pinch of salt
55g/2oz/⅓ cup of grated root ginger
55g/2oz/⅓ cup of chopped stem ginger
55g/2oz/½ cup of glacé mango
1 tablespoon of fresh lemon juice

2 tablespoons of liquid skimmed milk
6 generous tablespoons of golden syrup (corn syrup) from a warmed spoon
1 medium free-range egg white

23cm/9 inch non-stick baking tin, lined with baking parchment (wax paper)

Preheat the oven to 190°C/375°F/Gas Mark 5

Place the oats, sugar, milk powder and salt in a bowl and mix them together. Stir in the grated ginger and stem ginger, followed by the mango, lemon juice and milk. Lastly, add the syrup and blend it all together.
Whisk the egg white until foamy but not stiff, then fold it into the dry mixture.
Spoon the mixture into the prepared tin and press it down firmly, especially around the sides.
Bake for about 25 minutes until golden brown and firm.
Leave the flapjacks to cool slightly before cutting into slices or triangles.

Rainbow Tarts

This is a special request from a little boy in Scotland who finds children's tea parties a sad affair because he can not eat wheat or nuts, so there are several recipes in this section just for him.

Makes 18

PASTRY
200g/7oz/scant 1 ½ cups of (WF) flour
55g/2oz/½ cup of sifted icing (confectioners') sugar
A pinch of salt
100g/3½oz/7 tablespoons of (DF) margarine
1 large free-range egg

FILLING
About a teaspoon of different coloured jam (jelly), for best effect, for example, raspberry, apricot, gooseberry, blackberry

3 x 6-hole non-stick bun trays, each lined with a circle of baking parchment (wax paper)

Preheat the oven to 180°C/350°F/Gas mark 4

Make the pastry by mixing all the ingredients together in a food processor briefly but just enough to gather the dough into a ball.

Roll out the pastry on a floured board, cut into large enough circles to fit your bun trays and press a pastry circle into each hole.

Choose a variety of jam (jelly) and place a spoonful of the selected jam (jelly) into the centre of each tart.

Bake the jam (jelly) tarts for 20 minutes or until the pastry is golden.

Cool the tarts in the trays and then ease them out and onto a wire rack.

Store in an airtight container until needed.

Little Apple Tarts

I always keep a jar of apple purée in the cupboard because it is marvellous for instant tarts, mousses and sauces.

Makes 18

PASTRY

200g/7oz/scant 1 1/2 cups of (WF) flour
55g/2oz/1/2 cup of sifted icing (confectioners') sugar
A pinch of salt
100g/3 1/2oz/7 tablespoons of (DF) margarine
1 large free-range egg

FILLING

12 heaped tablespoons of organic ready-made apple
   purée (sweetened with honey)
3 large free-range egg yolks
Freshly grated nutmeg
1/2 teaspoon of ground cinnamon
1/2 teaspoon of (GF) mixed (pie) spice
1 small dessert apple, peeled, quartered, cored
   and sliced very thinly
A little lemon juice

3 x 6-hole non-stick bun trays, each lined with a circle
   of baking parchment (wax paper)

Preheat the oven to 180°C/350°F/Gas mark 4

Make the pastry by mixing all the ingredients together in a food processor briefly but just enough to gather the dough into a ball.

Roll out the pastry on a floured board and cut into large enough circles to fit your bun trays.

Press each pastry circle into the prepared trays.

Mix the apple purée and egg yolks in a bowl with a little grated nutmeg, cinnamon and mixed (pie) spice. Prepare the apple and brush each slice with a tiny amount of lemon juice.

Place about three quarters of a tablespoonful of the apple purée into the centre of each tart.

Decorate with one slice of the apple, pressed slightly into the purée.

Bake the tarts for 30 minutes, or until the apple is just browned at the edges, the filling is set and the pastry golden.

Cool in the trays and then ease them out and onto wire racks. Eat on the day of baking or keep in the refrigerator so that they do not go soggy.

Children's Cup Cakes

Baking with the help of children in the kitchen is always fun and very messy – this is no exception!

Makes 12

130g/4½oz/½ cup plus 1 tablespoon of (DF) margarine, softened

130g/4½oz/½ cup plus 1 tablespoon of caster (superfine) sugar

2 large free-range eggs

125g/4½oz/generous ¾ cup of (WF) flour

1 teaspoon of pure Madagascan vanilla extract

2 heaped teaspoons of (GF) baking powder

A choice of food colourings, according to taste

Icing (confectioners') sugar, sifted (about 200g/7oz/1⅓ cups in total)

12 glacé cherries or angelica slices or silver balls (check they are all suitable)

12-hole, non-stick bun tray, lined with paper cases

Preheat the oven to 200°C/400°F/Gas mark 6

Beat the margarine and the sugar together until light and fluffy in the food processor. Transfer the mixture to a bowl and fold in the eggs and flour half at a time. Gently fold in the vanilla and baking powder.

Divide the mixture between the paper cases and cook for 12–15 minutes, or until golden brown. Cool the cup cakes on a wire rack.

Now make the icing. You can make several different coloured icings by mixing a few drops of pink, yellow or green food colouring to suit your decoration. For example, pink icing with the cherries and yellow icing with angelica or green icing with silver balls.

Stir the icing (confectioners') sugar with the chosen colour and a little water in a small bowl until the icing is thick and smooth. Do not make it runny or the icing will drip off the cakes.

Spread the icing on each cake and decorate. Leave the icing to set before devouring the cakes. Store any that are left in an airtight container.

Spanish Orange Cake

You can make a chocolate orange cake with this recipe by replacing 4 tablespoons of the ground almonds with the same amount of cocoa powder. Dust with cocoa powder mixed with icing (confectioners') sugar for decoration.

Serves 6

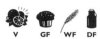

3 large sweet oranges
255g/9oz/1¼ cups of caster (superfine) sugar
6 large free-range eggs, separated
340g/12oz/4 cups of ground almonds
2 teaspoons of ground cinnamon
A pinch of salt

Icing (confectioners') sugar and ground cinnamon
   to decorate
1 packet of cinnamon sticks

A deep-sided 23cm/9-inch round loose-bottomed
   cake tin, greased with a little sunflower oil and lined
   with baking parchment (wax paper)

Preheat the oven to 180°C/350°F/Gas mark 4

Put the whole, unpeeled oranges in a heavy-based pan and cover with cold water. Bring slowly to the boil and simmer for 2 hours, topping up with more water if necessary. Drain the oranges and leave to cool for 20 minutes. Cut the oranges in half and discard any pips.

Liquidize the oranges in a food processor with the sugar, egg yolks, almonds and ground cinnamon. Transfer the mixture to a large mixing bowl.

In a separate bowl, whisk the egg whites and salt until stiff, but not dry. Gradually fold in the orange mixture with a metal spoon. Spoon into the prepared cake tin and bake for 1½ hours, or until the cake is firm to the touch.

Leave to cool in the cake tin and then turn out onto a plate.

Mix some cinnamon with icing (confectioners') sugar, and dust the cake with it. Serve, decorated with a little bundle of cinnamon sticks in the centre of the cake.

Double Sticky Gingerbread

Cakes baked with treacle (molasses) or honey will last for weeks in a tin, so are useful for big families.

Serves 6

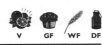

V GF WF DF

115g/4oz/³/₄ cup of rice flour
100g/3¹/₂ oz/²/₃ cup of buckwheat flour
1 teaspoon of bicarbonate of soda (baking soda)
1 tablespoon of ground ginger
1 tablespoon of ground (GF) mixed (pie) spice
1 teaspoon of crushed cardamom seeds
100g/3¹/₂ oz/7 tablespoons of (DF) margarine
55g/2oz/¹/₄ cup of soft brown sugar

130g/4¹/₂ oz/¹/₃ cup of black treacle (molasses)
130g/4¹/₂ oz/¹/₃ cup of golden syrup (corn syrup)
2 large free-range eggs, beaten
200ml/7fl oz/³/₄ cup of natural soya yogurt (or goat's
  yogurt, which is not DF)

19cm/7¹/₂ inch square cake tin, greased and lined with
  baking parchment (wax paper)

Preheat the oven to 170°C/325°F/Gas mark 3

Sift the flours, bicarbonate of soda (baking soda), ginger, spice and cardamom seeds together in
a mixing bowl.
Put the margarine, sugar, treacle (molasses) and syrup into a saucepan and warm over a low heat
until the treacle and syrup have melted and the sugar has dissolved.
When the mixture has cooled, beat in the eggs. Pour this mixture into the flour. Add the yogurt
and beat with a wooden spoon to a smooth batter. Pour the batter into the prepared tin and bake
for 1¹/₄ hours. Cool for 15 minutes in the tin and then transfer to a wire rack. When cold, store in
an airtight container until needed.

Cranberry Date Loaf

Cranberry Date Loaf is delicious on its own or lightly buttered. You can use whatever dried fruit you happen to have.

Makes about 10 slices

70g/2¹/₂oz/¹/₃ cup of dried cranberries

70g/2¹/₂oz/¹/₃ cup of dried cherries

70g/2¹/₂oz/¹/₂ cup of dried chopped dates

125ml/4fl oz/¹/₂ cup of hot black china tea

The grated rind of 1 orange

3 tablespoons of orange juice

140g/5oz/²/₃ cup of pear or apple purée, unsweetened

140g/5oz/1 cup of potato flour

100g/3¹/₂oz/²/₃ cup of rice flour

1 heaped teaspoon of cream of tartar

1 teaspoon of bicarbonate of soda (baking soda)

140g/5oz/²/₃ cup of (DF) margarine

100g/3¹/₂oz/1 generous cup of ground almonds

70g/2¹/₂oz/1 cup of flaked almonds

1 free-range egg, beaten

70g/2¹/₂oz/¹/₂ cup of carrot, grated

2 teaspoons (GF) mixed (pie) spice

1kg/2.2lb loaf tin, greased and lined with baking parchment (wax paper)

Preheat the oven to 180°C/350°F/Gas mark 4

Mix the fruit with the boiling hot tea, orange rind and juice in a bowl and leave to cool.
Add the fruit purée and blend in.
In another bowl, sift the flours and mix in the cream of tartar and bicarbonate of soda (baking soda). Then, using a blunt-ended knife, mix in the margarine until it resembles crumbs. Add the ground almonds and half the flaked almonds, the fruit with its liquid, egg, carrot and spice.
Spoon into the prepared tin and sprinkle with the remaining flaked almonds.
Cover loosely with foil and bake for 50 minutes or until an inserted skewer comes out clean.
Cool and turn out onto a rack until cold. Serve in slices.

Banana and Lemon Iced Loaf

Overripe bananas needn't go to waste again. You can whip up this cake and freeze it if no one is around to appreciate it!

Serves 6

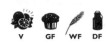

140g/5oz/1 cup of rice flour
140g/5oz/1 cup of buckwheat flour
3 heaped teaspoons of (GF) baking powder
½ teaspoon of salt
255g/9oz/1 cup plus 2 tablespoons of (DF) margarine
255g/9oz/1¼ cups of sugar

650g/23oz of bananas, peeled and mashed
4 large free-range eggs
4 tablespoons sifted icing (confectioners') sugar
½–1 tablespoon lemon juice

23–25cm/9–10 inch loaf tin, greased and lined

Preheat the oven to 180°C/350°F/Gas mark 4

Sift the flours into a bowl with the baking powder and salt.
In a food processor, beat the margarine, sugar and bananas together until smooth, then briefly blend in the eggs. Stir this into the flour mixture until it is evenly blended.
Pour into the loaf tin and bake for about 1–1¼ hours or until an inserted skewer comes out clean and the cake is just firm. If it browns too quickly, cover the tin loosely with foil.
Cool in the tin for 10 minutes and then transfer to a wire rack to cool.
Mix the icing (confectioners') sugar with enough of the lemon juice to make a thick enough paste. When the cake is cold, drizzle the icing over the top. Store the cake in an airtight container until needed.

Chocolate and Cinnamon Birthday Cake

Try using novelty chocolates to decorate this enticing birthday cake. A very good selection of dairy-free and gluten-free chocolates is available from the mail order company listed on page 264.

Serves 10–20

CAKE

550g/1lb 3oz of (DF/GF) plain chocolate, broken
    into pieces
310g/11oz/1⅓ cups of (DF) margarine
2 teaspoons of ground cinnamon
600ml/20fl oz/2½ cups of boiling water
400g/14oz/2 cups of caster (superfine) sugar
3 large free-range eggs, beaten
200g/7oz/scant 1½ cups of rice flour
200g/7oz/scant 1½ cups of millet flour
3 teaspoons of (GF) baking powder
1 teaspoon of bicarbonate of soda (baking soda)

CAKE ICING

300g/10½oz/2 cups of icing (confectioners')
    sugar, sifted
75ml/2½ fl oz/¼ cup of orange liqueur or brandy
    (alternatively for children use weak coffee)
100ml/3½ fl oz/⅓ cup of soya cream

PIPING ICING

A dash of boiling water to melt 2 heaped tablespoons
    of (DF/GF) cocoa powder
140g/5oz/1 cup of sifted icing (confectioners') sugar
140g/5oz/⅔ cup of (DF) margarine

Candles or novelty chocolates to decorate

24.5cm/9½ inch, loose-bottomed, spring-form,
    round cake tin, greased and lined with baking
    parchment (wax paper)
30cm/12 inch round silver paper cake board

Preheat the oven to 170°C/325°F/Gas mark 3

Make the cake first. Place 350g/12oz/2 cups of the chocolate in a bowl with 225g/8oz/1 cup of the margarine, the cinnamon and the boiling water, and carefully melt in the microwave. Stir until smooth, then stir in the sugar and beaten eggs.
Fold in the flours, the baking powder and bicarbonate of soda (baking soda) very briefly. Spoon the mixture into the prepared tin and bake in the centre of the oven for 50 minutes, or until the centre of the cake is just firm. (An inserted skewer should come out clean.) Leave the cake to cool down in the tin and then remove it from the tin onto a wire rack to cool completely.

Make the cake icing by heating the remaining 200g/7oz/1¼ cups of chocolate with the remaining 100g/3½oz/7 tablespoons margarine in a bowl in the microwave. Stir in the icing (confectioners') sugar, liqueur and soya cream, and beat until smooth and blended.

Place the cake on the centre of the cake board and spread it all over with the icing. Use a palette knife for a clean finish and work quickly as the icing sets pretty fast.

Make up the piping icing. (For a smooth and light icing, ensure that the boiling water just makes the cocoa melt.) Put all the piping icing ingredients together in a food processor and beat until smooth and just soft enough to pipe around the cake.

Fill a clean piping bag fitted with a rosette or shell-style nozzle with the piping icing and carefully pipe rosettes or shells all around the base and top of the cake.

Decorate the cake when the icing has set, according to the age of the recipient – candles or chocolates!

Blackberry and Apple Cake

I devised this fat-free cake recipe for some American friends of mine staying in London for a while. You can substitute any kind of dried berry for the blackberries when they are not in season or are too expensive to buy. The apples are also delicious substituted with pears in season.

Serves 10

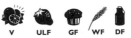

200g/7oz/2 cups of peeled, cored and chopped
   eating apple
170g/6oz/1 cup of finely grated carrot
255g/9oz/2¼ cups of fresh or frozen blackberries
240ml/8fl oz/1 cup of cranberry juice
140g/5oz/1 cup of buckwheat flour
140g/5oz/1 cup of maize flour
3 teaspoons of (GF) baking powder
A pinch of salt

1 teaspoon of ground cinnamon
2 teaspoons of (GF) mixed (pie) spice
2 large free-range egg whites, lightly beaten
170g/6oz/1 cup of soft (light) brown sugar, sifted

1kg/2.2lb non-stick loaf tin, lined with baking
   parchment (wax paper)

Preheat the oven to 180°C/350°F/ˉGas mark 4

Place the apple, carrot, blackberries and cranberry juice in a non-stick saucepan, bring to the boil, then set aside to cool.

Sift the flours, baking powder, salt and spices into a bowl. In separate bowl, whisk the egg whites until stiff, then gradually whisk in the sugar until you have a stiff meringue.

Stir the fruit mixture into the flour mixture and then fold in the meringue. Spoon the mixture into the prepared baking tin and gently smooth over the top.

Bake in the oven for about 1½ hours, or until the loaf is well risen and golden brown. An inserted skewer should come out clean when the cake is cooked through.

Leave the cake to cool, then turn it onto a wire rack and remove the paper. When the cake is completely cold, wrap it in foil and store in an airtight container until needed.

Cranberry and Orange Angel Cake

I use my heart-shaped cake tin for this light sponge. Soaked in liqueur and piled high with raspberries, this unbelievably easy cake is delicious for those of us on a low-fat diet.

Serves 12

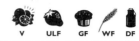

115g/4oz/¾ cup of rice flour

285g/10oz/1½ cups of caster (superfine) sugar

10 medium free-range egg whites at room temperature

Generous ½ a teaspoon of (GF) cream of tartar

1 tablespoon of orange liqueur

100g/3½oz/½ cup of cut, dried mixed peel

70g/2½oz/½ cup of dried and sweetened cranberries

½ teaspoon of ground cinnamon

1 teaspoon of caster (superfine) sugar

A heart-shaped or standard non-stick angel cake tin, lined with baking parchment (wax paper)

Preheat the oven to 180°C/350°F/Gas mark 4

Sift together the flour and 100g/3½ oz/¾ cup of the caster (superfine) sugar into a bowl. In another bowl, beat the egg whites until foamy, add the cream of tartar and beat until they form soft peaks.

Beat 2 tablespoons at a time of the remaining sugar into the egg whites, until you have used up all the sugar and the meringue is glossy and stiff. Now fold in the liqueur and the mixed peel. Carefully sprinkle a little of the flour mixture over the meringue and gently fold it in. Continue this process until all the flour has been incorporated.

Spoon the meringue mixture into the prepared tin and sprinkle the cranberries over the top. Bake the cake for about 35 minutes, or until golden (an inserted skewer should come out clean if the cake is cooked through).

Allow the cake to cool a little in the tin, before turning out onto a wire rack. Mix the cinnamon with the caster (superfine) sugar and sprinkle over the cake. Set aside to cool completely.

The cake is best eaten fresh on the day. It can also be served as a pudding with a large bowl of luscious red berries and a pool of thick seasonal fruit sauce.

Passion Cake

I have absolutely no idea why carrot cakes are often called passion cakes but perhaps the idea of carrots seems too worthy and off-putting! Whatever the reason this passion cake is delicious.

Serves 8–10

240g/8¹/₂oz/1³/₄ cups of (WF) flour
500g/17oz/2¹/₂ cups caster (superfine) sugar
2 heaped teaspoons of (GF) baking powder
2 heaped teaspoons of ground cinnamon
240ml/8fl oz/1 cup of corn oil
3 large free-range eggs, beaten
2 teaspoons of pure Madagascan vanilla extract
455g/1lb/3¹/₄ cups of carrots (peeled weight),
   cooked and puréed
115g/4oz/1 cup of chopped walnuts
85g/3oz/1 cup of desiccated (shredded) coconut
170g/6oz/³/₄ cup of canned crushed pineapple, drained
85g/3oz/¹/₂ cup of plump sultanas (golden raisins)

SOFT ICING AND FILLING

250g/9oz/1 cup plus 2 tablespoons of (DF) margarine
400g/14oz/3 cups of icing (confectioners') sugar
Grated zest and juice of 1 small orange
1 tablespoon of orange liqueur
1 tablespoon of orange flower water
4 tablespoons of toasted coconut pieces

2 x 23cm/9 inch non-stick cake tins, lined with baking
   parchment (wax paper)

Preheat the oven to 180°C/350°F/ Gas mark 4

Sift the flour, sugar, baking powder and cinnamon into a bowl. Add the oil, eggs and vanilla extract and beat well. Fold in the carrots, walnuts, coconut, pineapple and sultanas (golden raisins).

Divide the batter evenly between the two prepared tins. Bake the cakes for about an hour or until the edges have come away from the sides of the tins and the cake is firm.

Leave the cakes to cool in the tins, then turn onto wire racks, remove the paper and let them get completely cold.

Make the icing by beating the margarine with the icing (confectioners') sugar until light and fluffy. Beat in the orange zest, orange juice and liqueur until smooth. Carefully beat in the orange flower water. The icing should be soft and light but you have to beat in all the ingredients a little at a time to avoid curdling the icing. If it begins to separate, quickly add more icing (confectioners') sugar and beat until smooth.

Place one cake on a serving plate and spread the one third of the filling over it, then cover the filling with the remaining cake. Decorate the cake with the remaining two thirds of the filling, spreading it lightly all over the cake.

Sprinkle the toasted coconut all over the cake and keep it in a cool place until ready to serve.

Lemon Curd Cake

This lovely cake is perfect for a serene English afternoon tea under an old shady tree.

Serves 6–8

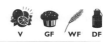

V GF WF DF

LEMON CURD

4 large lemons with good skins
8 large free-range egg yolks, beaten
100g/3½oz/7 tablespoons of (DF) margarine
340g/12oz/1²⁄₃ cups of caster (superfine) sugar

CAKE

170g/6oz/³⁄₄ cup of (DF) margarine
170g/6oz/1 cup less 2 tablespoons of caster
  (superfine) sugar
3 large free-range eggs
Grated zest of 1 large lemon

Juice of ½ a lemon
100g/3½oz/²⁄₃ cup of rice flour, sifted
70g/2½oz/½ cup of maize flour, sifted
2 teaspoons of (GF) baking powder

LEMON ICING

Zest of 1 lemon
Juice of ½ a lemon
140g/5oz/1 cup of icing (confectioners') sugar, sifted

A deep-sided 23cm/9inch non-stick, round cake tin,
  lined with baking parchment (wax paper)

Preheat the oven to 180°C/350°F/Gas Mark 4

First make the lemon curd. Grate the zest of the 4 lemons, then squeeze the juice and put both ingredients into a non-stick saucepan on extremely low heat. Add the lightly beaten eggs, margarine and sugar, and stir until sugar has dissolved. Continue cooking until the lemon curd thickens. Pour the lemon curd into clean, hot, dry jam (jelly) jars and seal. Cool and refrigerate the lemon curd and use within 4 weeks.

To make the cake, cream the margarine and sugar in a food processor until pale and fluffy. Transfer the mixture to a large bowl and beat in the eggs, a little at a time, with the zest and juice. Gently fold in the flours and baking powder. Spoon the batter into the prepared tin, smooth the top and bake for 25 minutes. Cool the cake slightly, then ease it out of the tin and peel off the paper. When the cake is cold, slice it in half horizontally, place the base of the cake on a serving plate and spread it with plenty of lemon curd. Cover with the other half of the cake.

Finally, mix all the ingredients for the lemon icing to a smooth, thick paste and drizzle over the top.

Keep the cake in the refrigerator until needed, but serve at room temperature.

If you don't want to make lemon icing, dust the cake with icing (confectioners') sugar only or sprinkle over the squeezed juice and seeds or 3–4 ripe passion fruit and then dust with icing (confectioners') sugar. Scrumptious also with blueberries, strawberries or raspberries on top and dusted with icing (confectioners') sugar.

Orange Cake with Marshmallow Topping

This recipe, given to me by some American friends, suits all ages and seasons. The exact weight of the three eggs in the recipe determines the amount of sugar, margarine and flour needed.

Serves 8–10

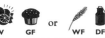

The same weight of:

3 large free-range eggs (in their shells); caster (superfine) sugar; (DF) margarine; and (GF) flour – rice flour and maize flour or millet flour, (WF) flour or barley flour, or any of the above flours in equal parts

Grated zest and juice of 2 large oranges

2 heaped teaspoons of (GF) baking powder

70g/2¹/₂oz/1¹/₂ cups of miniature marshmallows or ordinary marshmallows halved

225g/8oz/1¹/₂ cups of icing (confectioners') sugar, sifted

A deep-sided 20cm/8 inch non-stick, round cake tin, greased and lined with baking parchment (wax paper)

A long skewer for securing the cake

Preheat the oven to 190°C/375°F/Gas mark 5

First make the cake. Blend the sugar and margarine in a food processor until light and fluffy. Add three quarters of the orange juice and zest, and blend briefly. Add half the flour and mix briefly. Break the whole eggs into a bowl and whisk with a fork. Now add half the egg to the mixture in the food processor and whizz briefly. Add the remaining egg and whizz again. Briefly mix in the remaining flour and the baking powder.

Spoon the mixture into the prepared tin, bake for 15 minutes, then reduce the oven temperature to 180°C/350°F/Gas mark 4 and bake for another 15 minutes, or until well risen, golden and firm to touch.

Leave the cake to cool for 10 minutes in the tin, then turn out onto a plate. Peel off the baking parchment (wax paper) and leave the cake to stand, upside down, for 10 minutes.

Carefully tip the cake, so it is topside up, onto a serving plate.

Slice the cake in half horizontally, cover with marshmallows, then immediately cover the marshmallows with the remaining layer of cake.

Secure the cake by inserting a long skewer through the centre of the cake. Set aside to allow the warm cake to melt the marshmallows.

Now make the icing by gradually mixing the remaining orange juice and zest into a bowl of the sifted icing (confectioners') sugar and beating until smooth. You may not need all the juice, so add a little at a time.

Spread the icing over the cake (having removed the skewer) and chill it until it is set.

Serve the cake at room temperature but cover and return to the refrigerator for storage – if there is any left!

Dark Ginger Cake

I love really sticky gingerbread, so this is perfect. It is very useful for picnics or packed lunches as it does not crumble and has no icing or filling which can attach itself to anybody or anything.

Serves 8

140g/5oz/¹/₂ cup plus 2 tablespoons of (DF) margarine

140g/5oz/³/₄ cup of dark Mauritian sugar

2 large free-range eggs

115g/4oz/³/₄ cup of rice flour

115g/4oz/³/₄ cup of potato flour

285g/10oz/³/₄ cup of black treacle (molasses)

100g/3¹/₂oz/²/₃ cup of plump sultanas (golden raisins)

2 heaped teaspoons of ground ginger

100g/3¹/₂oz/¹/₂ cup of chopped stem ginger

1 tablespoon of ginger wine

1 teaspoon of bicarbonate of soda (baking soda)

23cm/9 inch square cake tin, greased and lined with baking parchment (wax paper)

Preheat the oven to 170°C/325°F/Gas mark 3

In a food processor, beat the margarine and sugar together until pale and creamy. Transfer to a large bowl, beat in the eggs and then add the flours, black treacle (molasses), sultanas (golden raisins), ground ginger and chopped ginger. Add the wine and bicarbonate of soda (baking soda) and mix thoroughly.

Put the mixture into the prepared tin and bake for about 1 hour. Reduce the heat to 150°C/300°F/Gas mark 2, cover the ginger cake with greased baking parchment (wax paper) and bake for another 45 minutes.

Leave the cake in the tin for 20 minutes and then turn out, upside down onto a wire rack to cool. When the cake is cold, peel off the baking parchment (wax paper), wrap the ginger cake in foil and store in an airtight container for up to a week.

Apple Cake

In England all sorts of irresistible apples are grown and we should all make more use of the wide choice available. Sadly most ancient varieties have been lost but some survive which date back to Anglo-Saxon times and retain their original 14th-century names.

Serves 8

V   GF   WF   DF

130g/4½oz/generous ¾ cup of rice flour

130g/4½oz/generous ¾ cup of millet flour

A pinch of salt

2 teaspoons of (GF) baking powder

55g/2oz/⅔ cup of ground almonds

100g/3½oz/½ cup of caster (superfine) sugar (plus
   1 tablespoon extra)

200g/7oz/1 cup less 2 tablespoons of (DF)
   margarine

455g/1lb/4 cups dessert apples, peeled and cored,
   half roughly chopped for inside the cake and half
   sliced for the top of the cake

2 large free-range eggs, beaten

2 tablespoons of cider or apple juice

40g/1½oz/3 tablespoons of brown sugar

1 teaspoon of ground cinnamon

55g/2oz/½ cup of flaked almonds

23cm/9 inch square cake tin, oiled and lined with
   baking parchment (wax paper)

Preheat the oven to 180°C/350°F/Gas mark 4

First, sift the flours, the salt and baking powder into a large bowl and stir in the ground almonds and caster (superfine) sugar. Add 170g/6oz/¾ cup of the margarine and rub in with your fingertips until the mixture resembles breadcrumbs.

Stir in the roughly chopped apples and beaten eggs. Add the cider and then spoon the mixture into the tin. Neatly arrange all the sliced apples on top and sprinkle with 1 tablespoon of caster (superfine) sugar.

Bake for 45 minutes, or until the cake is just firm and the apples well browned. If the apples start to burn, cover the cake loosely with foil until the cake is just cooked through.

Meanwhile, heat the rest of the margarine, the brown sugar and the cinnamon together in a pan until it dissolves. Stir in the flaked almonds.

Take the cake out of the oven and spread with the almond mixture. Return it to the oven to bake for a further 10 minutes, or until an inserted skewer comes out clean.

Leave the cake in the tin for 30 minutes, then turn out on to a serving plate and remove the baking parchment (wax paper). Serve the cake cold.

Honey and Rosewater Roll

This is also delicious filled with (DF) vanilla ice-cream and crushed raspberries or strawberries and served immediately with a soft fruit purée.

Serves 10

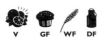

ROLL

4 large free-range eggs, separated

115g/4oz/generous ¾ cup of icing (confectioners')
   sugar and extra for sprinkling

1 tablespoon of rosewater

55g/2oz/scant ½ cup of rice flour

55g/2oz/scant ½ cup of potato flour

1 teaspoon of (GF) baking powder

FILLING

3 tablespoons of scented runny honey

1 teaspoon of rosewater

100g/3½oz/7 tablespoons of (DF) margarine

100g/3½oz/¾ cup of icing (confectioners') sugar,
   sifted

Raspberry jam (jelly)

A clean tea towel

33 x 23cm/13 x 9 inch non-stick Swiss roll/ roulade
   tin, completely lined with one piece of baking
   parchment (wax paper)

Preheat the oven to 190°C/375°F/Gas mark 5

First make the roll. In a large bowl, beat the egg whites with an electric whisk until they form soft peaks. Gradually sift and fold in half the icing (confectioners') sugar until the mixture stands in firm peaks.

In another bowl, beat the egg yolks and the remaining icing (confectioners') sugar until very thick. Stir in the rosewater. Gently fold in the flours and baking powder.

Lightly fold in the egg whites using a metal spoon, a third at a time, until all the egg whites are used up.

Lightly spread the mixture into the prepared tin and bake for 12 minutes until firm and springy when touched.

Sift and sprinkle the extra icing (confectioners') sugar onto a clean tea towel. Turn the cake onto the tea towel and carefully pull off the baking parchment (wax paper).

Cut any crisp edges off the cake, then roll up the cake in the tea towel and leave until it is cold.

Now make the filling. Beat the honey, rosewater, margarine and icing (confectioners') sugar together until smooth and spreadable (I usually use the food processor).

Carefully unroll the cake and spread it with as much or as little of the jam (jelly) as you like. Lightly spread the filling over the raspberry jam (jelly) and roll up the cake. Transfer the cake to a serving plate and dust it with extra sifted icing (confectioners') sugar.

Earl Grey Tea Loaf

This is a delightfully old-fashioned fruit loaf and as it improves with a few days in the cake tin, it is ideal for busy weekend entertaining or picnics.

Serves 8

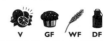

140g/5oz/²⁄₃ cup of (DF) margarine

170g/6oz/generous ³⁄₄ cup of caster (superfine) sugar

240ml/8fl oz/1 cup of strong Earl Grey tea

255g/9oz/1½ cups of dried mixed fruit, glacé pineapple, cherries, sultanas (golden raisins) or raisins

100g/3½oz/²⁄₃ cup of rice flour

100g/3½oz/²⁄₃ cup of potato flour

2 teaspoons of (GF) baking powder

Finely grated zest and juice of 1 lemon

1 large free-range egg, beaten

70g/2½oz/²⁄₃ cup of coarsely chopped walnuts

A little demerara sugar for sprinkling

25 x 10cm/10 x 4 inch loaf tin, greased and lined on the base

Preheat the oven to 180°C/350°F/Gas mark 4

Put the margarine, sugar, tea and fruit in a saucepan, bring slowly to the boil and simmer for 5 minutes, stirring occasionally. Remove the saucepan from the heat and, when the mixture is cool, sift the flours and baking powder into the fruit mixture and mix it all together. Fold in the lemon zest and juice, the beaten egg and walnuts.

Pour the mixture into the prepared tin, sprinkle with the demerara sugar and bake for about 1–1½ hours, until well risen and firm in the centre. Leave the loaf in the tin to cool, then turn out onto a wire rack to cool.

Store in an airtight container until needed. Serve the loaf sliced.

Fruit Cake

This recipe makes two fruit cakes so that one can be frozen for another time. If you are entertaining lots of people then you can make this as one large fruitcake, which will take an extra hour to cook.

Serves 10 (each small cake), or 20 (1 large cake)

V   GF   WF   DF

1kg/2.2lb/7 cups of mixed dried fruit such as sultanas (golden raisins), currants, mixed peel, glacé cherries and pineapple

100ml/3½ fl oz/⅓ cup of Amaretto di Saronno liqueur

300ml/10fl oz/1¼ cups of orange juice

100ml/3½ fl oz/⅓ cup of coconut cream

Grated zest of 1 orange

6 large free-range eggs, separated

225g/8oz/1 generous cup of dark brown soft sugar

140g/5oz/⅔ cup of unsweetened canned chestnut purée

225g/8oz/1 cup of (DF) margarine, softened

115g/4oz/1⅓ cups of ground almonds

115g/4oz/¾ cup of rice flour

70g/2½oz/½ cup of whole blanched almonds to decorate (or more for a more luxurious look)

2 x 20cm/8-inch square non-stick cake tins at least 9cm/3½ inch deep, lined with baking parchment (wax paper)

Kitchen foil

Preheat the oven to 170°C/325°F/Gas mark 3

If you have time, it is a great idea to macerate the fruit 24 hours in advance. To do this, put all the dried fruit, Amaretto, orange juice and coconut cream together in a very large bowl with the grated orange. Mix well to blend the liquids and coat the fruit. Cover the bowl and keep in a cool place until needed.

To make the cake, put the egg yolks, soft brown sugar, chestnut purée and margarine in the food processor and blend until fluffy. Transfer to a very large bowl. Sift the ground almonds and the rice flour into the mixture and fold in. Stir in the prepared dried fruit and all the liquid.

Whisk the egg whites in a bowl until they are stiff and then fold them into the fruit mixture.

Divide the mixture between the 2 tins and decorate with the whole almonds.

Bake in the oven for 2½ hours or until the cakes are firm and cooked all the way through. You will probably need to cover the cakes with foil half way through the cooking so that the cakes do not burn. If the sides seem to be getting too dark then wrap foil around the tins as well and cook for a little longer to make sure the centre is cooked through.

Leave the cakes to cool in the tins and then turn them out and remove all the paper.

Serve the cakes when they are cold and then store in an airtight container until needed.

Macadamia Nut Pound Cake

Make this cake the day before you need it so that the flavours have time to develop.

Serves 8

70g/2¹/₂oz/¹/₂ cup of macadamia nuts
Extra rice flour
70g/2¹/₂oz/¹/₂ cup of polenta (maize)
130g/4¹/₂oz/generous ³/₄ cup of rice flour
1 heaped teaspoon of (GF) baking powder
¹/₂ teaspoon of bicarbonate of soda (baking soda)
A pinch of salt
140g/5oz/1 cup of icing (confectioners') sugar

130g/4¹/₂oz/¹/₂ cup plus 1 tablespoon of (DF) margarine
2 large free-range eggs, beaten
100ml/3¹/₂ fl oz/¹/₃ cup of goat's or sheep's yogurt
3 tablespoons of maple syrup

A deep-sided 23cm/9 inch round or square, loose-bottomed, non-stick cake tin, greased and lined with baking parchment (wax paper)

Preheat the oven to 190°C/375°F/Gas mark 5

Put the nuts on a non-stick baking sheet and cook them in the oven until golden. Roughly chop the nuts and sprinkle with a little bit of extra rice flour.

Sift together the polenta (maize), flour, baking powder, bicarbonate of soda (baking soda) and salt into a large bowl.

Beat the icing (confectioners') sugar and margarine in a food processor until pale and fluffy.

Add the eggs and half the flour mixture and mix briefly. Add the yogurt, maple syrup, nuts and the rest of the flour mixture and blend very briefly.

Spoon into the prepared cake tin and bake for 40 minutes, or until brown and firm to touch. (An inserted skewer should come out clean when the cake is cooked.)

Leave the cake to cool in the tin, then peel off the baking parchment (wax paper) and leave the cake to go cold on a wire rack.

Wrap the cake in clingfilm (plastic wrap) or keep it in an airtight container until needed.

Marsala and Pecan Cake

This is very much a grown-up cake, the sort you get at afternoon tea in a smart London hotel. However, if you are not a tea drinker then a double espresso and a slice of this cake is a real treat at any time of the day.

Serves 8–12

CAKE

4 large free-range eggs, separated and 1 extra egg
    white
140g/5oz/³⁄₄ cup of caster (superfine) sugar
200g/7oz/1³⁄₄ cups of pecan nuts
4 heaped tablespoons of 100% rye breadcrumbs or
    (GF) breadcrumbs
¹⁄₂ a heaped teaspoon of cream of tartar

MARSALA ICING

225g/8oz/1 cup of (DF) margarine, softened
255g/9oz/1³⁄₄ cups of icing (confectioners') sugar,
    sifted
75ml/2¹⁄₂ fl oz/¹⁄₄ cup of Marsala
Pecan halves to decorate
(GF) cocoa powder to dust

A deep-sided 20cm/8 inch non-stick, loose-bottomed
    cake tin, greased and lined with baking parchment
    (wax paper)

Preheat the oven to 180°C/350°F/Gas mark 4

Beat the egg yolks and sugar together in the food processor until pale and fluffy. Add the nuts and process briefly, so that they are finely chopped. Add the breadcrumbs and mix together for a moment. Transfer the mixture into a large bowl.

In another bowl, beat the egg whites with the extra egg white and the cream of tartar until stiff. Fold 2 tablespoons of the egg whites into the pecan mixture and then gently fold in the rest. Spoon the mixture into the cake tin and bake for about 35 minutes, or until firm and brown and well risen.

Leave the cake to cool in the tin for 20 minutes, then turn it out and peel off the baking parchment (wax paper). Allow the cake cool on a wire rack.

Now make the icing. Beat the margarine and icing (confectioners') sugar until light and fluffy in the food processor, then carefully add a little Marsala at a time. Do not over beat or it will separate, also take care not to add too much Marsala as this will also make it separate.

Slice the cake in half horizontally and when it is cold, spread the sponge with about one third of the icing. Cover with the top of the cake and spread the rest of the icing all over the cake.

Decorate the top of the cake with pecan halves and dust with sifted cocoa powder.

Store in an airtight container in the refrigerator until needed.

Coconut and Lime Cake

This light summery cake tastes fresh and zingy, just what I love on a hot summer's day with a glass of iced tea and lemon.

Serves 8–10

CAKE

170g/6oz/³/4 cup of (DF) margarine, softened
170g/6oz/generous ³/4 cup of caster (superfine) sugar
Grated zest of 2 limes and their juice
4 large free-range eggs, separated
100g/3¹/2oz/²/3 cup of rice flour, sifted
100g/3¹/2oz/²/3 cup of millet flour, sifted
Pinch of salt
1 heaped teaspoon of (GF) baking powder
55g/2oz/²/3 cup of desiccated (shredded) coconut
240ml/8fl oz/1 cup of goat's or sheep's natural yogurt
¹/2 teaspoon of cream of tartar

ICING

3 ripe passion fruit, halved and flesh scooped into a bowl
Juice of ¹/2 a lime
170g/6oz/1¹/4 cups of sifted icing (confectioners') sugar or more if the mixture is too runny

A deep-sided 23cm/9 inch, non-stick, loose-bottomed cake tin, greased and lined with baking parchment (wax paper)

Preheat the oven to 180°C/350°F/Gas mark 4

Beat the margarine and sugar in a food processor, then beat in the lime zest and egg yolks. Transfer the mixture to a bowl and fold in the flours with the salt, baking powder and coconut. Fold in the lime juice and yogurt. Whisk the cream of tartar with the egg whites until stiff in another bowl. Fold the egg whites into the cake mixture and spoon into the prepared cake tin.
Bake in the oven for about 45 minutes, or until golden brown, firm and springy to touch.
Cool the cake in the tin for 10 minutes, then turn out and peel off the baking parchment (wax paper). Leave the cake to cool on a wire rack.
Meanwhile, make the icing. Mix the passion fruit pulp with the lime juice and beat in the icing (confectioners') sugar using a wooden spoon. Add more icing (confectioners') sugar if the icing is too runny (this will depend on the size of passion fruit and lime you are using and how ripe and juicy they are).
Place the cake on a serving plate and spread the icing over the top of the cake. Leave to set in a cool place. Keep the cake in an airtight container in the refrigerator until needed.

Rhubarb and Orange Cake

It had never occurred to me to use rhubarb in a cake so I was astonished when I saw a recipe for one. Cinnamon, rhubarb and nuts are remarkably good together and it is an excellent way of using up leftover rhubarb.

Serves 8–12

V   GF   WF   DF

CAKE

255g/9oz/1³⁄₄ cups of washed, trimmed and dried
  rhubarb, cut into 4cm/1¹⁄₂ inch lengths
200g/7oz/1 cup of caster (superfine) sugar
Finely grated zest and the juice of 1 orange
140g/5oz/²⁄₃ cup of (DF) margarine, softened
2 large free-range eggs
85g/3oz/9 tablespoons of rice flour
1 teaspoon of (GF) baking powder
100g/3¹⁄₂oz/1 cup of desiccated (shredded) coconut
1 teaspoon of ground cinnamon

TOPPING

30g/1oz/2 tablespoons of (DF) margarine
30g/1oz/2 tablespoons of caster (superfine) sugar
85g/3oz/³⁄₄ cup of slivered (flaked) almonds
1 teaspoon of ground cinnamon

A deep-sided 20cm/8 inch loose-bottomed,
  non-stick cake tin, greased and lined with baking
  parchment (wax paper)

Preheat the oven to 180°C/350°F/Gas mark 4

Put the rhubarb into a bowl with 55g/2oz/¹⁄₄ cup of the sugar, the orange zest and juice. Mix well and then cook in the microwave for about 4 minutes, or until the rhubarb is just cooked and all the juices have seeped out.

Drain the rhubarb in a sieve and keep the juice for something else as it is too good to waste!

In another bowl, beat the margarine and the remaining sugar together until light and fluffy. Stir in the eggs, flour, baking powder, coconut and cinnamon as lightly and quickly as possible.

Mix the rhubarb into the cake mixture and transfer to the prepared tin. Bake in the oven for about 40 minutes until well browned and fairly firm.

Meanwhile, melt all the topping ingredients together in a saucepan and stir over very low heat until the nuts are evenly coated.

Take the cake out of the oven and spread the nut mixture over the top of the cake.

Return the cake to the oven and bake for another 20 minutes. The cake should now be firm and springy to touch.

Leave the cake to cool in the tin for about 1 hour and then turn it onto a wire rack and remove the baking parchment (wax paper).

Serve in thick chunks and store any leftovers wrapped in clingfilm (plastic wrap) in an airtight container.

Walnut and Chocolate Cake

This is hugely indulgent and wicked! A double bonus of chocolate in the cake and in the icing as well. This is particularly suitable for chocolate indulgence at Easter.

Serves 8

V   GF   WF   DF

CAKE

140g/5oz/²/₃ cup of (DF) margarine, softened
140g/5oz/³/₄ cup of caster (superfine) sugar
2 large free-range eggs, beaten
100g/3¹/₂oz/²/₃ cup of rice flour, sifted
30g/1oz/¹/₃ cup of ground almonds
Pinch of salt
1 heaped teaspoon of (DF/GF) baking powder
85g/3oz of (DF/GF) dark chocolate, coarsely chopped
   or grated
115g/4oz/1 ¹/₃ cups of walnut halves, as fresh as
   possible, roughly chopped
1 tablespoon of strong black coffee

ICING

100g/3¹/₂oz of (DF/GF) dark continental chocolate
30g/1oz/2 tablespoons of (DF) margarine
85g/3oz/1 cup of walnut halves, as fresh as possible

A deep-sided 20cm/8 inch square, loose-bottomed
   non-stick cake tin, greased and lined with baking
   parchment (wax paper)

Preheat the oven to 180°C/350°F/Gas mark 4

Cream the margarine and sugar in a food processor until pale and fluffy. Gradually add the eggs, flour, almonds and salt, mixing only very briefly. Transfer the mixture to a large bowl and fold in the baking powder, chopped chocolate, chopped walnuts and coffee.
Spoon the mixture into the prepared tin and bake for 30 minutes, or until firm to the touch. Cool the cake for 15 minutes in the tin and then lift it out, remove the base with the baking parchment (wax paper) and place it on a wire rack until cold. Peel the baking parchment (wax paper) off the sides of the cake.
Melt the chocolate for the icing with the margarine in a small bowl in the microwave and stir it until it is smooth.
Spread the icing over the top of the cake and once it has set, arrange the whole walnut halves all over the cake.
Cut the cake into squares or bars and keep it in an airtight container until needed.

Banana and Chocolate Loaf

This is ideal for picnics, as it slices up very easily and keeps well in foil. The only fat comes from the grated chocolate but it is so minimal, a mere 1g per slice! The loaf tastes even better the day after it was made.

Serves 10

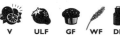

2 medium-sized, very ripe bananas, peeled
200ml/7fl oz/³/4 cup of pure apple juice
60ml/2fl oz/¹/4 cup of lemon juice
140g/5oz/1 cup of buckwheat flour
140g/5oz/1 cup of maize flour
3 teaspoons of (GF) baking powder
A pinch of salt
2 large free-range egg whites

140g/5oz/scant 1 cup of soft (light) brown sugar
30g/1oz/¹/3 cup of coarsely grated (DF/GF) dark chocolate
2 teaspoons of pure chocolate extract (fat-free)

1kg/2.2lb non-stick loaf tin, lined with baking parchment (wax paper)

Preheat the oven to 180°C/350°F/Gas mark 4

In a small bowl, mash the bananas, apple juice and lemon juice together until completely blended.
Sift together the flours, baking powder and salt in a separate bowl.
In another bowl, beat the egg whites until stiff, then gradually whisk in the sugar.
Add the grated chocolate and chocolate extract to the banana mixture and stir the mixture into the dry ingredients. Now quickly fold in the meringue.
Spoon the loaf mixture into the prepared tin and gently smooth over the top. Bake the loaf for 1 hour or until it is firm. (An inserted skewer should come out clean when the loaf is cooked through.)
Cool the loaf in the tin, then turn it out onto a wire rack and remove the paper.
When the loaf is cold, wrap in foil and store in an airtight container until needed.

Easter Simnel Cake

This traditional Easter cake is not served at any other time of the year. I have never come across it anywhere other than England. Apparently, the 11 balls of marzipan signify the 11 Apostles of Jesus – Judas was not counted.

Serves 8–16

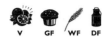

170g/6oz/³/4 cup of (DF) margarine

170g/6oz/generous ³/4 cup of caster (superfine) sugar

3 large free-range eggs and 1 extra egg white

115g/4oz/³/4 cup of rice flour

115g/4oz/³/4 cup of maize flour

Pinch of salt

1 heaped teaspoon of ground cinnamon

1 teaspoon of freshly grated nutmeg

100g/3¹/2oz/¹/2 cup of glacé cherries, cut into quarters

55g/2oz/¹/3 cup of cut mixed peel, chopped

255g/9oz/1³/4 cups of currants

100g/3¹/2oz/³/4 cups of sultanas (golden raisins)

Finely grated rind of 1 lemon

Lemon juice if necessary

500g/1lb 1oz of ready-to-roll (GF) marzipan

130g/4¹/2oz of ready-to-roll (GF) marzipan, for the 11 decorative balls

Baking parchment (wax paper) and string

18cm/7 inch round cake tin, greased and lined with baking parchment (wax paper)

Ribbon to decorate the cake

Preheat the oven to 150°C/300°F/Gas mark 2

Beat the margarine and sugar in a food processor until fluffy. Transfer the mixture to a large bowl. In another bowl, lightly whisk the 3 whole eggs, then gradually beat them into the creamed ingredients.

Sift the flours, salt and spices over the surface and fold into the mixture using a metal spoon. Add all the fruit and the lemon rind, folding together to give a smooth dropping consistency. If the mixture is too firm, add a little more lemon juice.

Divide the 500g/1lb 1oz marzipan in half. Lightly dust a surface with the icing (confectioners') sugar and roll out one half to a 16cm/6¹/2 inch circle.

Spoon half the cake mixture into the prepared tin. Place the round of marzipan on top and cover with the remaining cake mixture. Press down gently with the back of a spoon to level the surface. Tie a double thickness of baking parchment (wax paper) round the outside of the tin. Bake in the oven for about 2¹/2 hours. When it is cooked the cake should be a rich brown colour and firm to the touch. Cool in the tin for about 1 hour and then turn it out. Ease off the baking parchment (wax paper) and leave to cool completely on a wire rack.

Roll the remaining marzipan into a 16cm/6¹/2 inch circle.

Lightly beat the egg white in a small bowl and brush a little of it over the top of the cake.

Place the circle of marzipan on top of the cake and crimp the edges with your fingertips.

Use the 125g/4¹/₂oz of marzipan to make 11 small balls. Use the palm of your clean hands to make the balls smooth and even.

Fix the 11 balls around the top edge of the cake with a little more of the beaten egg white.

Brush the marzipan with the remaining egg white and place under a hot grill (broiler) for 1–2 minutes until the marzipan balls are well browned.

Tie a ribbon around the cake and store in an airtight container for up to a week.

Christmas Cake

The longer this cake is kept the more succulent it will be, but do store it for at least a month. Baste with brandy from time to time and keep wrapped in foil, in an airtight container.

Serves 20

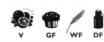

V   GF   WF   DF

CAKE
500g/17oz/3½ cups of raisins
400g/14oz/3 cups of dried currants
140g/5oz/1⅓ cups of dried pineapple, chopped
140g/5oz/¾ cup of glacé cherries
140g/5oz/1 cup of dried figs, chopped
140g/5oz/¾ cup of candied citrus peel, chopped
170g/6oz/1¼ cups of white rice flour
200g/7oz/1½ cups of brown rice flour
¼ teaspoon of salt
½ teaspoon of (GF) mixed (pie) spice
1 teaspoon of grated nutmeg
2 teaspoons of ground allspice
370g/13oz/1½ cups of (DF) margarine

370g/13oz/1¾ cups of brown sugar
6 large free-range eggs
6 tablespoons of brandy

ICING
4–5 tablespoons of smooth apricot jam (jelly)
Icing (confectioners') sugar for rolling
500g/17oz of (GF) golden marzipan
1kg/2.2lb of ready-made-to-roll (GF) white icing
Ribbon, decorations or food colouring (optional)

25cm/10 inch cake tin, greased and lined with a
   double layer of baking parchment (wax paper)
(DF) sunflower margarine

Preheat the oven to 150°C/300°F/Gas mark 2

Put the fruit in a bowl and cover with boiling water. Leave until tepid, then drain.
Sift the flours with the salt, mixed (pie) spice, nutmeg and allspice. Cream the margarine and sugar together in a large bowl until soft and light (or use a food processor and then return the mixture to the bowl). Add 1 egg at a time, beating it into the mixture. When you have added all the eggs, mix in the flour mixture in several batches. Finally, add the brandy and dried fruits. Lightly grease the paper in the cake tin with the (DF) sunflower margarine, then spoon the batter into the tin and smooth the top, hollowing the centre slightly. Bake for 3 hours or until cooked through. (Insert a skewer into the cake – it is ready if the skewer comes out clean. Test in several places.) If the cake browns too quickly cover loosely with foil.
Leave to cool in the tin and then unmould and peel off the paper. Wrap the cake in foil and store. The week you intend to eat the cake, unwrap it and place on a cake board. Gently heat the apricot jam (jelly) and brush it all over the cake. Sprinkle a work surface with icing (confectioners') sugar and roll out the marzipan and cover the cake with it. Trim off any excess and press closely into the cake. Trim again if necessary. Leave for 24 hours in a cool place to dry out. Roll out the ready-made icing in the same way, cover and trim. Decorate and store in an airtight container.

Wedding Cake

This is the cake that we made for my wheat- and dairy-free wedding. It had elegant white icing, so to give it some extra decoration we wrapped the cake in beautiful gold ribbon and finished it with a bouquet of perfect white roses on the top. It was very simple and effective and was admired by everyone at the reception.

Serves 100–150 guests

V   GF   WF   DF

If you want to have traditional columns and tiers, ornate icing and decoration, I suggest that you make the cake, let it mature and cover it with the marzipan. Then take it to an expert and have it professionally iced, decorated and delivered to your reception.

EQUIPMENT

3 square cake tins: 32cm/12½ inch; 25cm/10 inch; 16.5cm/6½ inch
1 × 41cm/16-inch-square silver paper cake board
2 matching smaller square silver paper cake boards with about 2.5cm/1 inch spare border around both cakes
White, gold, silver or coloured silk ribbon of your choice
Fresh or silk flowers, or other suitable decoration for the top of the cake
Baking parchment (wax) paper and tin foil to line the tins, extra (DF) margarine for greasing
Icing equipment if you need it (piping bags, nozzles etc.) – do not attempt to ice your cake unless you know that you are brilliant at it!
9 white columns to support the cakes

CAKE

1.5kg/3.3lb/10 cups of raisins
1kg/2.2lb/7 cups of dried currants
500g/17oz/3 cups of dried pineapple, chopped
600g/1lb 5oz/7 cups of glacé cherries, halved
500g/17oz/3 cups of dried figs, chopped
400g/14oz/4½ cups of candied citrus peel, chopped
250g/8½oz/1¾ cups of stoned (pitted) dates, chopped
600g/1lb 5oz/4½ cups of rice flour

600g/1lb 5oz/4½ cups of millet flour
1 teaspoon of salt
2 tablespoons of (GF) mixed (pie) spice
1 tablespoon of grated nutmeg
2 tablespoons of ground allspice
1 tablespoon of ground cinnamon
1.1kg/2lb 6oz/4¾ cups of very soft (DF) sunflower margarine and extra for greasing paper
1.2kg/2lb 10oz/6 cups of brown sugar
20 large free-range eggs
24 tablespoons of brandy
255g/9oz/2 cups of whole blanched almonds, roughly chopped
Grated rind of 2 oranges

CAKE COVERING

A standard-sized jar of smooth apricot jam (jelly)
4 × 500g/17oz packets of ready-made to roll (GF) golden marzipan
Extra icing (confectioners') sugar for rolling

ICING

This is the icing recipe that I used, but most traditional royal icing recipes will be gluten and dairy free so these could be used as an alternative if you prefer.

4 medium free-range egg whites
800g/1lb 12oz/5½ cups of (GF) white icing (confectioners') sugar, sifted
1 tablespoon of lemon juice
1 teaspoon of glycerine

Preheat the oven to 150°C/300°F/Gas mark 2

First make the cakes. Pour just enough boiling water over all the fruit in 2 huge bowls. Leave until the fruit becomes tepid. Drain and set the bowls of fruit to one side.

Meanwhile, grease and line the three cake tins with a double layer of baking parchment (wax paper) and then grease the paper for extra protection.

Sift the flours with the salt, mixed (pie) spice, nutmeg, allspice and cinnamon into another huge bowl.

In another enormous bowl, bucket or jam (jelly) pan, cream together the margarine and sugar until soft and light.

Add 4 eggs at a time to this margarine mixture until you have added all the eggs. Now, gently mix in the flour and spices. Finally, add the brandy, dried fruits, nuts and grated orange rind.

Spoon this batter into the prepared cake tins and smooth over the tops, hollowing the centres slightly to prevent the cake rising and splitting in the centre.

Wrap double layers of foil around the outside of each cake tin and loosely cover the top of the cakes with foil. This will help to prevent the sides and top of the cake from burning while the centre of the cake is still undercooked.

Now begin baking (allow up to 6 hours baking time if you are planning to go out for the evening, that way none of the cakes will be hurried and undercooked).

Bake the largest cake for at least 4 hours or until an inserted skewer comes out clean from the centre of the cake (this could be as much as 5 hours if your oven is not as hot as mine is!). The second size cake should take about 3 hours, and the smallest cake should take about $1\frac{1}{2}$ hours (test both with a skewer as before – test them all in several places for reliability).

Leave the cakes to cool in their tins for 24 hours, then remove the cakes from the tins and peel off the baking parchment (wax paper). Wrap the cakes in foil and store in airtight containers for at least 2 weeks, but preferably for 2 months, before the wedding. Choose a cool place to let the cakes develop and mature nicely

A week before the wedding, unwrap the cakes and place them in the centre of their corresponding sized silver boards. Make sure they are in the centre as you won't be able to move them later!

The cakes are now ready to be covered in jam (jelly). Gently heat the apricot jam (jelly) in a bowl in the microwave and then brush the jam (jelly) all over the top and sides of the cakes. This seals the cakes and holds down the marzipan.

Now marzipan the cakes. (I used 2 blocks of marzipan to cover the large cake, $1\frac{1}{4}$ blocks for the middle size cake and $\frac{3}{4}$ of a block for the smallest cake. The marzipan was not too thick but was not so thin that you could see the dark fruit underneath.) Sprinkle a work surface with icing (confectioners') sugar and roll out each block of marzipan with a rolling pin. When it is the correct thickness, use the rolling pin to lift the marzipan over the whole cake (the marzipan will stick to the jam (jelly) immediately so make sure you aim accurately).

If you can not cover the cake with one piece of marzipan, roll out smaller pieces to fill in any part of the cake that is not covered. You can mould it gently with your fingers so that it all blends in together and looks nice and smooth. It is most important to cover the cake completely so that the fruit will remain moist.

Trim off any excess marzipan and press closely to the cake. Trim again if necessary. Leave the cake for 24 hours to dry out in a cool place.

Repeat this with the remaining two cakes.

After 24 hours, when all three cakes will be ready, you can start icing the base cake first, or take the cakes to be iced and decorated.

FOR EACH BATCH OF ICING (You will need three batches for the whole cake and may need a fourth if you are doing ornate decoration)

Beat the egg whites until slightly frothy in a food processor. Add the icing (confectioners') sugar, lemon juice and glycerine and beat until smooth. Transfer the icing to a bowl and keep covered until needed, but do use it as quickly as you can.

Ice the cake. Make up the icing (1 batch at a time) and spread over each cake so that they are completely covered with icing and perfectly smooth and even all over.

Leave them to set hard before starting to decorate the cake. (Remember to wipe clean the silver boards before the icing sets.)

When the icing is completely hard and set, make up a final batch of icing for the decoration and pipe your chosen design on to the cakes (you can add a little colour to the batch of icing you use for decorating the cake, if you wish, pale pink, pale blue or pale yellow can be used, but I kept mine all white).

Once all the icing has set, take the cake to the reception and assemble it. Put 1 column in the centre of the largest cake and then 4 more columns, positioned to support the middle size cake, on top of the base cake. Repeat with the remaining 4 columns to support the smallest cake on top of the middle cake.

Finally, decorate the cakes with flowers and ribbons. Don't forget the cake knife!

Chocolate Truffles

These truffles could not be easier to make and are such a treat for birthdays, Christmas and Easter. Serve them in little gold paper cases with coffee after dinner parties or just spoil yourself when you have a lust for chocolate!

Serves 10 (2 each)

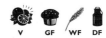

255g/9oz of (DF/GF) luxury dark chocolate
55g/2oz/¹/4 cup of (DF) margarine
75ml/2¹/2fl oz/¹/4 cup of soya cream

Brandy, Cognac or Cointreau (or 1 teaspoon of pure Madagascan vanilla extract and 1 teaspoon of warm water or black coffee, if no alcohol is desired)
(DF/GF) cocoa powder

Break the chocolate into a bowl, add the margarine and melt briefly in the microwave.
Stir in the cream and mix well together. Add the brandy or liqueur, or the vanilla extract and coffee mixture, and stir together until smooth.
Leave to cool and when the mixture is firm, mould teaspoons of the chocolate into balls in your hands. Roll the balls in cocoa powder and leave in the refrigerator to set.
(Alternatively, roll them in browned nuts and chill until needed.)
Place the truffles in little foil or paper cases and serve cool but not rock hard and cold.
You can arrange them in a pretty box, tied up with a ribbon to give as a gift – these truffles need to be kept chilled, so please ask the lucky recipient to keep them in the refrigerator until shortly before needed!

Fondant Cape Gooseberries

The sweet, fondant coating perfectly complements the small explosion of tart juices. You can dip the Cape gooseberries (physalis) in (DF) caramel or (DF/GF) luxury chocolate.

Serves 10 (4 each)

40 ripe Cape gooseberries (physalis)

140g/5oz/1 cup of sifted icing (confectioners') sugar

1 tablespoon of orange liqueur

1 tablespoon of freshly squeezed orange juice

A few drops of food colouring, optional

1 large plate or tray with about 2 tablespoons of sifted icing (confectioners') sugar sprinkled over it

Hold the stalks of the Cape gooseberries (physalis) and gently open out the papery lanterns that conceal the berries. Fold the wings right back, giving them a little twist as you do so.

In a small bowl, beat the icing (confectioners') sugar with the liqueur and orange juice until smooth. Stir in a couple of drops of food colouring if desired, or divide the mixture in half and colour one half, leaving the other plain.

Holding the wings of the fruit carefully, dip the berries into the icing until evenly covered.

Allow the excess to drip off before placing it on to the prepared plate or tray.

Keep in a cool place (not the refrigerator) and eat within 48 hours.

Chocolate-dipped Strawberries

The ultimate luxury must be the combination of fresh strawberries and bitter chocolate. A very sensual and easy pudding for St. Valentine's night, or an ideal treat for the calorie-conscious chocolate lover! For just two of you, halve the quantities in the recipe.

Serves 4 (5 each)

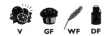

20 large ripe strawberries
140g/5oz of (DF/GF) luxury dark continental chocolate
A few drops of sunflower oil

A plate sprinkled with sieved (DF/GF) cocoa powder
Kitchen (paper) towels

Wash the strawberries and carefully dry them on kitchen (paper) towels.
Microwave the chocolate in a small bowl with a couple of drops of oil until just melted and then stir until smooth.
Dip the strawberries into the chocolate and let any excess chocolate drip off.
Place on the prepared plate and chill until needed.
Serve the strawberries on a glass or silver dish for special occasions and devour them within 48 hours.

Peppermint Creams

If you don't like chocolate but love peppermint these are perfect for you. They are so easy to prepare that children can make them as presents.

Makes lots!

455g/1lb/3 cups of icing (confectioners') sugar, sifted
1 teaspoon of lemon juice
2 teaspoons of water

1 large free-range egg white, lightly whisked
1 teaspoon of peppermint flavouring or oil
Green food colouring, optional

Mix the sugar with the lemon juice, water and enough egg white to make a pliable mixture. Divide the mixture in half and flavour one half with peppermint and a few drops of green food colouring and the other half with only the peppermint flavouring.

Knead on a clean surface, dusted with icing (confectioners') sugar, and then gently roll out each mixture separately into a long sausage.

Slice the dough into neat little rounds or form into balls and flatten slightly with the back of a fork.

Leave the peppermint creams somewhere safe and cool for 24 hours until thoroughly dry.

You can pack them into little paper cases and put them into a pretty box or keep the peppermint creams in an airtight container until needed.

Walnut and Pecan Creams

Another easy, though slightly more sophisticated recipe which children can make and give as presents.

Makes lots!

V GF WF DF

455g/1lb/3 cups of icing (confectioners') sugar, sifted
1 teaspoon of lemon juice
1 large free-range egg white, lightly whisked
1 dessertspoon of coffee essence
1 teaspoon of water

At least 12 whole walnut halves
At least 12 whole pecan halves
100g/3½oz (DF/GF) luxury dark continental
  chocolate, optional

Mix the icing (confectioners') sugar, lemon juice and egg white in a bowl until pliable. Add the coffee essence and water. Knead on a clean surface dusted with icing (confectioners') sugar. Shape the mixture into balls about 2.5cm/1 inch in diameter, press half a walnut into half of the coffee balls and press the pecans into the remaining coffee balls (this should flatten the balls slightly).

For chocolate-drizzled creams, melt the chocolate in a small bowl in the microwave, stir until smooth and drizzle over the nuts on each sweet.

Put the walnut and pecan creams into little paper cases and leave them for 24 hours to set and dry. Transfer to a pretty box or keep them in an airtight container until needed.

CHAPTER 11

Breads, Muffins and Scones

Cumin Seed and Rye Bread

This recipe makes 2 loaves so you can pop one into the deep freeze. You can use any sort of seeds that you like.

Makes 2 loaves

455g/16oz/3¼ cups of rye flour
310g/11oz/2¼ cups of white rice flour
1 teaspoon of salt
14g/½oz/1 package of (WF) easy-bake (instant) yeast
300ml/10fl oz/1¼ cups of unsweetened apple juice
  mixed in equal parts with warm water

2 tablespoons of black treacle (molasses)
1 tablespoon of cumin seeds

2 non-stick loaf tins, greased

Preheat the oven to 200°C/400°F/Gas mark 6

Sift together the flours and salt in a bowl. Mix in the yeast and make a well in the dry ingredients, then stir in the warm apple juice and water mixture.
Dip a tablespoon into boiling water to heat it and then use the spoon to add the treacle (molasses) to the warm mixture and mix until you have a firm dough.
Knead thoroughly on a lightly floured surface for 10 minutes. Divide the mixture between the 2 non-stick loaf tins, cover with clingfilm (plastic wrap), and leave in a warm place until the dough has doubled in size.
Place the tins on a baking sheet. Sprinkle the tops of the bread with a little water and then the cumin seeds. Bake in the oven for 45 minutes.
Remove from the oven to cool slightly before leaving on a wire rack to cool completely.
Serve cold in slices or freeze until needed.

Sun-dried Tomato and Coriander Seed Bread

This bread is delicious with soups and starters, and also makes wonderful sandwiches for picnics or your daily lunch box. For a change you can swap the tomatoes to chopped black olives or fried onions. Alternatively, use chopped, stoned (pitted) dates for a sweeter combination.

Makes 2 loaves

455g/1lb/3¼ cups of rye flour

310g/11oz/2¼ cups of (WF) flour

1 teaspoon of salt

14g/½oz/1 package of (WF) easy-bake (instant) yeast

300ml/10fl oz/1¼ cups of unsweetened apple juice, mixed with the same amount of warm water

2 tablespoons of black treacle (molasses)

2 tablespoons of finely chopped sun-dried tomatoes

1 tablespoon of coriander seeds

2 large non-stick loaf tins or 2 non-stick trays, greased

Extra flour for kneading dough

Preheat the oven to 200°C/400°F/Gas mark 6

Sift together the flours and the salt in a bowl. Mix in the yeast, then make a well in the dry ingredients and stir in the warm apple juice water mixture.

Dip a tablespoon into boiling water to heat it and then quickly use the spoon to add the treacle to the warm mixture. Mix until you have a firm dough. Remove the dough from the bowl and knead thoroughly on a lightly floured surface for 8 minutes.

Add the chopped tomatoes and knead the dough for another 2 minutes. Divide the mixture into the 2 non-stick loaf tins, or onto the 2 non-stick trays, cover the dough with clingfilm (plastic wrap) and leave in a warm place until the dough has doubled in size.

Place the dough in the tins on a baking sheet, sprinkle the bread tops with a little water and then gently press in the coriander seeds. Bake in the oven for about 35 minutes.

Allow the loaves to cool slightly, then turn out onto a wire rack to cool completely.

Serve the bread in slices and keep it fresh in sealed polythene bags.

Chilli and Herb Cornbread

This is a recipe from my American friend, Vicky Maggione, for corn bread and it can be used to accompany soups, casseroles and salads. To make a sweet bread, see the recipe on page 247.

Serves 6–8

V GF WF DF

70g/2½oz/½ cup of rice flour	120g/4oz/⅔ cup of either chopped sweetcorn
70g/2½oz/½ cup of maize flour/meal	kernels or chopped olives and sun-dried
140g/5oz/1 cup of instant polenta	tomatoes or 120g/4oz/⅔ cup of cooked chopped
1 tablespoon of (GF) baking powder	onion or bacon
¾ teaspoon of salt	1 mild chilli pepper, seeded and chopped
2 teaspoons of runny honey	1 tablespoon of chopped herbs, either thyme, parsley,
2 large free-range eggs	sage or chives
300ml/10fl oz/1¼ cups of soya milk	Poppy seeds to decorate
3 tablespoons of corn oil	
A few drops of (GF) chilli sauce/oil	A large loaf tin, greased and lined with baking
	parchment (wax paper)

Preheat the oven to 200°C/400°F/Gas mark 6

Sieve and mix the dry ingredients into a bowl.
In another bowl, whisk the honey, eggs, milk, oil and chilli sauce/oil with the chopped sweetcorn, or whatever you have chosen.
Add the chilli pepper and herbs and mix together well. Stir this into the flours.
Pour the batter into the prepared tin, sprinkle with poppy seeds and bake for 35 minutes, or until an inserted skewer comes out clean.
Serve in thick slices.

Southern Cornbread

Cornmeal makes glorious golden yellow bread that has a traditional American/Italian flavour seldom used in England. The bread is ideal for a delicious breakfast or as a tea bread.

Serves 8

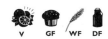

70g/2½oz/½ cup of rice flour

70g/2½oz/½ cup of maize flour

1 tablespoon of (GF) baking powder

140g/5oz/1 cup of quick-cook polenta (maize) or cornmeal

1 teaspoon of salt

340ml/12fl oz/1⅓ cups of apple juice

85g/3oz/6 tablespoons of (DF) margarine, melted

2 large free-range eggs, beaten

3 teaspoons of runny honey

200g/7oz/1¼ cups of pine nuts, toasted golden brown under the grill (broiler)

23cm/9-inch square, non-stick baking tin or a loaf tin, greased

---

Preheat the oven to 200°C/400°F/Gas mark 6

Sift together the flours and baking powder in a bowl. Stir in the polenta (maize) and salt and make a well in the centre of the flour.

Beat the apple juice and margarine together in another bowl. Whisk together the eggs and honey in a separate bowl. Add both mixtures to the flour mixture and stir thoroughly. Stir in the pine nuts and tip into the prepared tin.

Bake the cornbread for 30 minutes until well risen and golden brown. Allow the bread to cool, then turn it out onto a wire rack to cool completely.

Cinnamon, Honey and Oat Bread

This is a good emergency bread as I always have porridge oats at home but I often run out of the various kinds of flours needed for wheat-free bread.

Serves 8

V · WF · DF

7g/¹/₄oz/¹/₂ package of (WF) easy-bake (instant) yeast

1 teaspoon of salt

2 tablespoons of honey

400ml/14fl oz/1³/₄ cups of warm water

1 tablespoon of vegetable oil

500g/17oz/6 cups of porridge oats, processed finely
  to a flour

2 heaped teaspoons of ground cinnamon

1–2 tablespoons of sesame or sunflower seeds

2 greased non-stick loaf tins

Preheat the oven to 180°C/350°F/Gas mark 4

Place the yeast, salt and honey in a large bowl with the warm water and oil, and then mix in the processed oats and cinnamon.

Add the seeds and then knead with floured hands on a floured board for 10 minutes.

Divide the dough in two and shape to fit into the tins. Set aside to prove for about 30 minutes, allowing the dough to rise slightly. Bake for 1 hour or until the bread is firm.

Cool on a wire rack and then slice to serve.

Walnut Bread

I love sandwiches, but because of my wheat intolerance I can not buy them in the shops, so this is the food I have missed most. It is also the hardest snack to replace for speed and nutrition. Thankfully, I can now just slice up this loaf and freeze the slices in pairs ready for action!

Serves 8

14g/¹/₂oz/1 package of (WF) easy-bake (instant) yeast
1 teaspoon of salt
2 teaspoons of honey
400ml/14fl oz/1 ¾ cups of warm water
2 tablespoons of vegetable oil
500g/17oz/6 cups of porridge oats, processed
   to a fine flour

2 heaped teaspoons of ground cinnamon
A pinch of grated nutmeg
2 tablespoons of chopped walnuts

1 large non-stick loaf tin or non-stick baking tray,
   greased

Preheat the oven to 180°C/350°F/Gas mark 4

Put the yeast, salt and honey in a large bowl. Add the warm water and oil, then mix in the processed oats, cinnamon and nutmeg.

Knead the dough with floured hands on a floured board for 10 minutes. Divide the dough in half and briefly knead in the walnuts. Shape the dough into an oval and place it in the centre of the tray.

Leave the dough to prove in a very warm place for about 30 minutes, allowing it to rise slightly. Place the dough in either the loaf tin or on the baking tray and bake for 1 hour until the bread is firm. Cool the bread on a wire rack and when the bread is cold slice and serve.

Sesame Corn Crackers

These savoury biscuits are very handy for dips, and to accompany soups or salads. They are also ideal for nibbling along with drinks or cocktails.

Makes 20

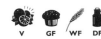

115g/4oz/²/₃ cup of quick-cook polenta
½ teaspoon of salt
340ml/12fl oz/1 ⅓ cups of boiling water
30g/1oz of melted (DF) margarine
1 teaspoon of sesame oil

A little (GF) chilli sauce/oil to taste
30g/1oz/¼ cup of sesame seeds

2–3 non-stick baking sheets, greased with a little
   margarine

Preheat the oven to 180°C/350°F/Gas mark 4

Put the polenta into a heatproof bowl with the salt and pour over the boiling water. Stir vigorously until it is smooth and then add the margarine, oil and chilli sauce/oil. It should be the consistency of thick cream. Add a little more water if necessary.

Spoon a tablespoon of the batter onto the sheet and spread into a circle. Make about 5 per sheet. Sprinkle with the seeds and bake in batches for about 20 minutes or until the edges are just brown and crispy.

Transfer them to wire racks until cool, crispy and ready to eat.

Crunchy Nutmeg and Banana Muffins

Mashed banana or grated carrot makes muffins extra moist and if you add (GF) muesli and nuts to the tops then you get a contrasting crunchy bite as well.

Serves 6

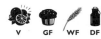

240ml/8fl oz/1 cup of sunflower oil

3 large free-range eggs

140g/5oz/³/4 cup of light muscovado sugar

1 large ripe banana, peeled and mashed

140g/5oz/1 cup of grated carrot

1 teaspoon of freshly grated nutmeg

100g/3¹/2oz/²/3 cup of rice flour

100g/3¹/2oz/²/3 cup of maize flour, sifted

2 teaspoons of (GF) baking powder

Demerara sugar for sprinkling

12-hole muffin tray, lined with paper muffin cases

Preheat the oven to 190°C/375°F/Gas mark 5

Beat the oil, eggs, muscovado sugar, mashed banana and grated carrot together and then gently mix in the nutmeg, the flours and the baking powder. Carefully spoon the mixture into paper cases in the muffin tray and sprinkle with demerara sugar.

Bake the muffins for 25 minutes, or until they are well risen and cooked through. Leave them to cool slightly in the paper cases and then serve them warm.

Date and Pecan Muffins

This is a lovely winter muffin – warming, sweet and filling to bolster you up for a cold morning.

Serves 6–12

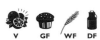

V   GF   WF   DF

170g/6oz/1¼ cups of rice flour
170g/6oz/1¼ cups of buckwheat flour
2 teaspoons of (GF) baking powder
1 teaspoon of bicarbonate of soda (baking soda)
140g/5oz/¾ cup of muscovado sugar
200g/7oz/1½ cups of dates, chopped
140g/5oz/1⅓ cups of chopped pecan nuts

1 heaped teaspoon of (GF) mixed (pie) spice
2 large free-range eggs
300ml/10fl oz/1¼ cups of apple juice
1 teaspoon of pure Madagascan vanilla extract
100g/3½oz/7 tablespoons of (DF) margarine, melted

12-hole muffin tray, lined with paper cases

Preheat the oven to 200°C/400°F/Gas mark 6

Sieve and then mix together all the dry ingredients. Add the dates, pecans and spice, and mix in. Beat the eggs, apple juice, vanilla extract and margarine together until frothy. Blend briefly into the flour mixture. Spoon into the paper cases and bake in the oven for 15–20 minutes until well risen and spongy to touch. Serve warm.

Corn and Blueberry Muffins

If you can't buy blueberries you can use bilberries or just swap around fruit to suit availability. You can also used dried fruit such as cranberries or cherries.

Serves 6–12

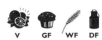

255g/9oz/1¾ cups of rice flour

2 teaspoons of (GF) baking powder

1 teaspoon of bicarbonate of soda (baking soda)

170g/6oz/1¼ cups of instant polenta

2 tablespoons of sugar

225g/8oz/1⅔ cups of frozen, fresh or dried blueberries

170g/6oz/¾ cup of soya yogurt with live ferments (or goat's yogurt, which is not DF)

2 tablespoons of lemon juice

The grated rind of 1 lemon

1 tablespoon of corn oil

255g/9oz/1¼ cups of crushed pineapple in natural juice, drained

Apple juice to moisten

12-hole, non-stick muffin tray, greased

Preheat the oven to 200°C/400°F/Gas mark 6

Sift the flour, baking powder and bicarbonate of soda (baking soda) into a bowl. Stir in the polenta, sugar and blueberries and mix thoroughly.
Mix the yogurt, lemon juice and grated rind, corn oil and crushed pineapple in another bowl. Pour the liquid into the dry ingredients and briefly stir in.
Add just enough apple juice to make the batter soft and easy to spoon into the moulds.
Place spoonfuls of the mixture into the tin and bake for about 15 minutes, or until golden brown and spongy to touch.
Leave the muffins in the tray for 5 minutes to cool and then transfer them to a wire rack until they are ready to eat.

Double Chocolate Chip Muffins

I have never quite managed to start the day with chocolate, but I have no doubts that to many people it is absolute bliss! However, for pure indulgence, these freshly baked muffins with a large cappuccino are heaven.

Serves 6

V   WF

140g/5oz/1 cup of rice flour
115g/4oz/³/4 cup of (WF) flour
1 heaped tablespoon of (DF/GF) cocoa powder
140g/5oz/³/4 cup of caster (superfine) sugar
1 tablespoon of (GF) baking powder
1 teaspoon of pure Madagascan vanilla extract
2 large free-range egg whites

140ml/5fl oz/²/3 cup of goat's yogurt
90ml/3fl oz/¹/3 cup of sweetened apple sauce
115g/4oz/²/3 cup of (DF/GF) chocolate chips or chopped dark chocolate

2 x 6-hole non-stick muffin trays, lined with paper muffin cases

Preheat the oven to 200°C/400°F/Gas mark 6

In a large bowl, stir together the first six ingredients. Make a well in the centre of the mixture.
In another bowl, beat the egg whites until foamy and then fold in the yogurt and apple sauce.
Add this mixture to the dry mixture and stir in the chocolate chips.
Spoon the batter into the tray of muffin cups, filling each one three-quarters full.
Bake the muffins for 20–25 minutes, or until an inserted skewer comes out clean.
Cool them in the tray for about 5–10 minutes before transferring to a wire rack to cool slightly.
Serve the muffins warm.

Date and Walnut Muffins

On a recent trip to America, we stayed in a hotel that had marvellous breakfasts. Baskets of warm and aromatic muffins full of fruit and spices lay waiting for us, how could we resist? We did not and it took me a long time to shed the pounds!

Serves 6

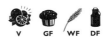

V   GF   WF   DF

115g/4oz/³/₄ cup of rice flour

115g/4oz/³/₄ cup of maize flour

2¹/₂ teaspoons of (GF) baking powder

¹/₂ fresh nutmeg, finely grated

1 heaped teaspoon of (GF) mixed (pie) spice

100g/3¹/₂oz/7 tablespoons of (DF) margarine, cut up into pieces

55g/2oz/scant ¹/₄ cup of caster (superfine) sugar

1 large free-range egg

300ml/10fl oz/1¹/₄ cups of natural soya yogurt (or sheep or goat's yogurt, which is not DF)

60ml/2fl oz/¹/₄ cup of water

170g/6oz/1 cup of chopped, stoned (pitted) dates

55g/2oz/¹/₂ cup of walnuts, chopped

Zest of 1 lemon

Demerara sugar for sprinkling

12-hole muffin tray, lined with paper muffin cases

Preheat the oven to 190°C/375°F/Gas mark 5

Sift the flours, baking powder and spices into a mixing bowl. Rub in the margarine with your fingertips until it resembles breadcrumbs, then stir in the sugar.

In another mixing bowl, beat the egg, yogurt and water together. Fold this mixture into the flour mixture using a metal spoon.

Add the chopped dates, walnuts and lemon zest and mix it all together.

Spoon the mixture into the paper cases in the muffin tray, sprinkle with demerara sugar and bake for 20 minutes, or until well risen and firm to touch.

Cool the muffins slightly in the paper cases and serve just warm.

Orange and Mincemeat Muffins

This is a great way to use up excess mincemeat left over from the Christmas and New Year festivities.

Serves 6

140g/5oz/1 cup of rice flour
140g/5oz/1 cup of maize flour
2¹/₂ teaspoons of (GF) baking powder
2 teaspoons of (GF) bicarbonate of soda
   (baking soda)
85g/3oz/6 tablespoons of dark muscovado sugar
1 teaspoon of ground cinnamon
A pinch of salt

300ml/10fl oz/1¹/₄ cups of natural soya yogurt (or
   sheep or goat's yogurt, which is not DF)
75ml/2¹/₂ fl oz/¹/₄ cup of fresh orange juice
Zest of 1 orange
4 tablespoons of sunflower oil
1 large free-range egg
255g/9oz/³/₄ cup of (GF) luxury mincemeat

12-hole muffin tin, lined with paper muffin cases

Preheat the oven to 200°C/400°F/Gas mark 6

Sift together the flours, baking powder, bicarbonate of soda (baking soda), sugar, cinnamon and a pinch of salt into a mixing bowl.
In another bowl, mix together the yogurt, orange juice and zest with the oil and egg.
Gently mix the wet ingredients into the dry ingredients using a metal spoon. Add the mincemeat and blend briefly.
Spoon the mixture into the paper cases in the muffin tray and bake for 20 minutes, or until golden and firm.
Leave the muffins to cool in the paper cases and serve them cold.

English Scones

The ultimate treat years ago when I could eat wheat, was to be invited by Rose, who did the PR for the Park Lane Hotel, to gossip like mad over a scrumptious afternoon tea in the very grand dining room there. Manners forgotten, every crumb of every scone was scooped up with clotted cream and strawberry jam (jelly) – all in the name of public relations of course!

Serves 6

V   WF

115g/4oz/³/₄ cup of rice flour
115g/4oz/³/₄ cup of barley flour
¹/₂ teaspoon of salt
1 tablespoon of caster (superfine) sugar
2 teaspoons of (GF) baking powder

55g/2oz/¹/₄ cup of (DF) margarine, cut up into pieces
1 large free-range egg, beaten
5 tablespoons of goat's milk
Extra goat's milk to glaze

Preheat the oven to 230°C/450°F/Gas mark 8

Preheat a baking sheet in the oven.
Sift the flours, salt, sugar and baking powder into a large bowl and rub in the margarine until the mixture resembles breadcrumbs. Make a well in the centre of the dry ingredients and stir in the beaten egg and goat's milk to make a soft dough.
Turn the dough out onto a floured surface and knead quickly and lightly to remove any cracks. Gently flatten the dough with the palm of your hand until it is about 2cm/³/₄ inch thick. Using a floured 5cm/2 inch cutter, cut out 5 dough rounds as close to each other as possible. If there are enough trimmings to make another one, then do so.
Carefully place all the rounds on the hot baking sheet and brush them with a little extra milk.
Bake in the centre of the oven for about 8–10 minutes or until they are firm, well risen and golden.
Cool the scones on a wire rack and serve them fresh with lots of jam (jelly)!

Walnut and Sage Scones

This is a very quick alternative to bread and makes up for not being able to eat things like pitta bread or the focaccia that I used to serve with soups. You can freeze the scones and reheat them briefly in the microwave for parties. They are delicious sprinkled with grated sheep's or goat's cheese, if you can tolerate dairy products.

Serves 8

115g/4oz/³/₄ cup of rice flour

100g/3¹/₂oz/²/₃ cup of buckwheat flour

55g/2oz/¹/₄ cup of (DF) margarine

¹/₄ teaspoon of (GF) chilli sauce/oil

100g/3¹/₂oz/1 cup of roughly chopped walnuts

15g/¹/₂oz/¹/₂ cup of chopped fresh sage leaves or
   1 tablespoon of dried sage leaves

1 egg and unsweetened apple juice to make the
   mixture up to 170ml/6fl oz/scant ³/₄ cup

2 teaspoons of (GF) baking powder

1 teaspoon of bicarbonate of soda (baking soda)

¹/₄ teaspoon of salt

A large baking sheet, greased and floured

Preheat the oven to 220°C/425°F/Gas mark 7

Sift the flours and mix with the margarine and chilli sauce/oil in a bowl. Rub gently with floured fingertips until the mixture resembles breadcrumbs and then add the walnuts and sage. Mix in well.

Beat the egg with the juice. Gently add the baking powder, bicarbonate of soda (baking soda) and salt to the walnut mixture. Quickly mix in the liquid and briefly knead into a dough.

Roll out on a floured board into a 3.5cm/1¹/₂ inch thick circle. Using a 5cm/2 inch cutter, cut out 8 scones and dust with flour or sprinkle with a suitable hard cheese if desired.

Bake for 10–15 minutes until brown and well risen.

Serve warm, or cool on a wire rack and freeze until needed.

Potato Scones

Years ago, when I cooked in a lodge at Balmoral Castle in Scotland during the fishing season, I was taught to make these griddle scones. I was told firmly never to use old mashed potatoes but to keep it for the salmon fishcakes we would be eating for breakfast every morning!

Serves 4

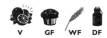

1 large potato or 255g/9oz peeled weight
30g/1oz/2 tablespoons of (DF) margarine
55g/2oz/scant 1/2 cup of rice flour
1/2 teaspoon of salt

1 teaspoon of (GF) baking powder
Some extra flour for sprinkling
A little oil

Peel the potato, cut it into chunks and cook in boiling water until tender.

Drain the potato in a colander until dry, transfer to a bowl and mash with the margarine until light and fluffy.

Sift the flour, salt and baking powder into a large bowl and mix in the mashed potato.

Roll the mixture into a ball and turn out onto a lightly floured board. Sprinkle flour on to the rolling pin and the dough and then roll out into a circle, about 5mm/1/4-inch thick.

Cut into 8 wedges and prick all over with a fork. Lightly grease a griddle or brush a frying pan (skillet) with oil and transfer the wedges to it as soon as it is hot.

Cook for 5 minutes on each side, until golden brown and firm.

Cool on a serving plate for 5 minutes before serving with (DF) margarine and a piping hot bowl of soup. For breakfast I suggest serving the potato scones with lashings of (DF) scrambled eggs and crispy bacon or poached eggs and ham.

Welsh Cakes

Now cooked on a griddle, these little Welsh gems would once have been cooked on a bakestone – a hot slab of stone over an open fire. Freshly cooked they need no embellishment, but once they are cold they do need a little butter or margarine.

Serves 6

GF / WF / DF

115g/4oz/³/4 cup of rice flour

115g/4oz/³/4 cup of millet flour

A pinch of salt

¹/2 teaspoon of (GF) mixed (pie) spice

¹/4 teaspoon of mace

55g/2oz/¹/4 cup of (DF) margarine

55g/2oz/¹/4 cup of white fat, cubed

85g/3oz/6 tablespoons of caster (superfine) sugar

85g/3oz/¹/2 cup of dried mixed fruit

1 free-range egg, beaten

1 tablespoon of apple or orange juice

Extra caster (superfine) sugar to sprinkle

Extra flour for rolling

A little oil

Sift the flours, salt and spices into a bowl. Rub in the margarine and white fat until you have a breadcrumb consistency. Stir in the caster sugar and dried mixed fruit, then mix in the egg and juice until you have a light dough.

Using a floured rolling pin, roll the dough out on a floured board until it is about 5mm/¹/4 inch thick, then use a 7.5cm/3 inch pastry cutter to cut out 12 rounds.

Lightly oil a griddle or a frying pan (skillet) and heat until hot.

Cook the cakes in batches for 4–5 minutes on each side until they are golden brown but still soft in the middle.

Sprinkle with caster (superfine) sugar when they are done and leave to cool slightly on wire racks until ready to eat.

Johnny Cakes and Maple Syrup

This was the height of our American breakfasts on our last visit to see my friends in Greenwich. I have adapted them and when we have time at the weekends, in between wading through piles of newspapers and colour supplements, we devour Johnny cakes with maple syrup and (DF) vanilla ice-cream – a huge sin in the book of calories!

Serves 4 (2 each)

V   GF   WF

140g/5oz/1 cup of fine (GF) corn meal or fine (GF) polenta (maize)

100g/3¹/₂oz/²/₃ cup of rice flour

4¹/₂ teaspoons of (GF) baking powder

2 teaspoons of caster (superfine) sugar

¹/₂ teaspoon of salt

2 large free-range eggs

300ml/10fl oz/1¹/₄ cups of goat's milk

30g/1oz/2 tablespoons of melted (DF) margarine

Oil for brushing the pan

Stir together the dry ingredients in a bowl.

Whisk the eggs and goat's milk in a large bowl. Gradually beat in the dry ingredients and, when well combined, stir in the melted margarine.

Heat two oiled griddle or non-stick frying pans (skillets) and use a tablespoon to drop the batter onto the very hot surface. Make the pancakes about 6cm/2¹/₂ inch in diameter.

Once the base is cooked and golden brown, turn the pancake over and cook the other side until they are cooked through.

Serve the pancakes straight from the griddle on heated plates with lots of maple syrup and your choice of (DF) margarine or butter.

My List of Ingredients

Lately, the biggest modern blight that disrupts social occasions is the ever-increasing list of foods to be avoided by children and adults of all ages. My recipes feature many familiar ingredients, but also staple foods such as soya products that you might normally hesitate to buy. The advantage of this list is that you will be able to whip up some little concoction at a moment's notice.

Cold pressed olive oil

Good quality sunflower and corn oil

Unsweetened apple juice and carrot juice

Jar of dairy-free pesto sauce and a jar of tahini

Ground almonds and other nuts

Cold pressed organic honey, treacle and
   golden syrup (corn syrup)

High quality sugar-free fruit jams (jelly)

Gluten-free chilli sauce/oil, soy sauce and
   Worcestershire sauce

Pure Madagascan vanilla extract

Dairy-free, gluten-free luxury dark chocolate

100% pure dairy-free, gluten-free cocoa powder

Soya milk, yogurt and cream

Tomor vegetarian margarine, dairy-free sunflower
   and soya margarine

Frozen dairy-free ice-cream dessert in different
   flavours (Swedish Glace or Toffuti are excellent)

Amaretto di Saronno liqueur, white rum and
   Cointreau

Marsala, dry white vermouth and Amaretto liqueur

Instant polenta (maize) and maize flour

Oats, buckwheat flour and rice flour

Gluten-free cornflour (cornstarch), potato flour,
   millet flakes and flour

Gluten-free baking powder and bicarbonate of
   soda (baking soda)

Gluten-free cream of tartar

Wild, arborio, brown, pudding and ground rice

Rice, corn and buckwheat spaghetti and pasta shapes

Large free-range eggs

Unrefined brown Mauritian sugar and caster
   (superfine) sugar

Icing (confectioners') sugar

All sorts of mixed dried fruits and pulses

Marigold yeast-free and gluten-free vegetable
   stock (bouillon) powder

Ground ginger and cinnamon

Gluten-free mixed (pie) spice – some brands
   contain gluten; if in doubt make up your own
   mixture with single spices

Coconut cream and milk

Frozen mixed berries

Fresh garlic, ginger, lemons and limes

Tofu

Jars of sweetened (with honey) apple purée

Sachets of powdered gelatine or vegetarian
   equivalent

Stem ginger in syrup

Gluten-free, ready-made-to-roll marzipan

100% pure maple syrup

Useful Addresses

ORGANIZATIONS

United Kingdom

Institute for Optimum Nutrition
Blades Court
Deodar Road
London SW15 2NU
Telephone 020 8877 9993

Action Against Allergy
24-26 High Street
Hampton Hill
Middlesex TW1 1PD
Telephone 020 8892 2711

Coeliac Society
PO Box 220
High Wycombe
Buckinghamshire HP11 2HY
Telephone 01494 437278

National Eczema Society
163 Evershalt Street
London NW1 1BU
Telephone 020 7388 4097

Myalgic Encephalomyelitis (ME) Society
PO Box 87
Stanford-le-Hope
Essex SS17 8EX
Telephone 01375 642466

British Heart Foundation
14 Fitzhardinge Street
London W1H 4DH
Telephone 020 7935 0185

IBS Network
Centre for Human Nutrition
Northern General Hospital
Sheffield S5 7AU
Telephone 0114 261 1531

Nutrition Associates
Galtres House
Lysander Close
Clifton Moregate
York YO3 OXB
Telephone 01904 691591

Berrydales Publishers
Berrydale House
5 Lawn Road
London NW3 2XS
Telephone 020 7722 2866
(*The Inside Story* food & health magazine)

The Vegetarian Society
Parkdale
Dunham Road
Altrincham
Cheshire WA14 4QG
Telephone 01619 280793

United States of America

Allergy Resources Inc.
PO Box 888
Palmer Lake
CO 80133
Telephone 800 873 3529

American Allergy Association
PO Box 7273
Menlo Park
CA 94026
Telephone 415 322 1663

American Celiac Society
Dietary Support Coalition
Ms Annette Bentley
58 Musano Court
West Orange
NJ 07052

Asthma and Allergy Foundation of America
1717 Massachusetts Avenue
Suite 305
Washington DC 20036
Telephone 202 265 0265

Gluten Intolerance Group
PO Box 23053
Seattle
WA 98102
Telephone 206 854 9606

STOCKISTS

United Kingdom

Wellfoods Gluten Free Flour
Wellfoods Ltd
Unit 6 Mapplewell Business Park
Mapplewell
Barnsley S75 6B
Telephone 01226 381712

The Fresh Food Company
326 Portobello Road
London W10 5RU
Telephone 020 8969 0351

Allergy Care
9 Coporation Street
Taunton
Somerset TA1 4AJ
Telephone 01823 325023

D&D Chocolates
261 Forest Road
Loughborough LE11 3HT
Telephone 01509 216400

Farm-a-round Ltd
(Organic fruit and vegetables delivered
to your door)
Forest House
4 Dartmouth Road
London SE23 3XU
Telephone 020 8291 4519

Glutano
(Gluten-free breads, cookies and pasta)
Unit 270 Centennial Park
Centennial Avenue
Elstree
Borehamwood
Herts WD6 3SS
Telephone 020 8953 4444

Provamel
Ashley House
86–94 High Street
Hounslow TW3 1NH
Telephone 020 8577 2727

The Village Bakery
(Gluten-free/wheat-free and yeast-free breads
delivered overnight)
Melmerby
Penrith
Cumbria CA10 1HE
Telephone 01768 881515

Growing Concern
(Organic rare-breed meats, bacon, ham and
poultry etc.)
Home Farm
Woodhouse Lane
Nanpanton
Loughborough
Leics LE11 3YG
Telephone 01509 237064

USA

Arrowhead Mills Inc.
(Mail order suppliers of grains, flours, legumes,
cereals and seeds)
Box 2059
Hereford TX 79045
Telephone 800 749 0730
Fax 806 364 8242

Bob's Red Mill Natural Foods Inc.
(Mail order stockists of grains, flours, legumes,
cereals and seeds)
5209 SE International Way
Milwauke
OR 97222
Telephone 503 654 3215
Fax 503 653 1339

Ener-g Foods Inc.
(Suppliers of food allergy products,
many rice-based, including rice flours, rice
pasta, egg substitute, almond milk mix as
well as baked goods)
PO Box 84487
Seattle
WA 98124-5787
Telephone 800 331 5222
Fax 206 764 3398

Gold Mine Natural Food Co.
(Stockist of rice, barley and other organic
grains and seeds)
3419 Hancock Street
San Diego
CA 92110-4307
Telephone 800 475 3663
Fax 619 296 9756

Jaffe Brothers Natural Foods
(Wholefood suppliers of nuts, nut butters,
dried fruits and grains)
PO Box 636
Valley Center
CA 92082 0636
Telephone 616 749 1133
Fax 619 749 1282

Mast Enterprises
265 North Fourth Street,
#616
Coeur D'Alene
ID 83814
Telephone 208 772 8213

Mountain Ark Trader
(Suppliers of grains and 100% buckwheat
noodles, Japanese-style silken tofu, soy
milk and rice milk)
PO Box 3170
Fayetteville
AR 72701
Telephone 800 647 8909
Fax 501 442 7191

Walnut Acres Organic Farms
Penns Creek
PA 17862
Telephone 800 433 3998
Fax 717 837 1146

Quick Reference Guide to Allergens

This quick reference guide will show you some of the ingredients that should be avoided by people suffering dairy, gluten or wheat intolerance.

Dairy	**Gluten**	**Wheat**
Butter	Durum wheat (pasta)	Wheat protein
Buttermilk	Barley	French garlic bread
Cheese	Semolina	Bread rolls
Cream	Sausages	Naan bread
Ghee	Malt	Yorkshire puddings
Hydrolysed whey protein	Oats	Noodles
Lactose	Wheat flour	Cakes
Margarine or shortening containing whey	Bran	Cookies
Milk solids	Prepared stuffing	Pancakes
Non-milk fat solids	Starch (including modified starch)	Scones
Skimmed milk powder	Rusk	Tortilla and nachos chips
Whey	Whisky	Monosodium glutamate
Yogurt	Beer	Prepared sandwiches
Ice-cream	Mixed (pie) spice	Prepared chilled soups
	Malt vinegar	Prepared chilled meals

As butter is tastier and may be healthier when heated than many margarines, I recommend using butter in place of margarine in the recipes if you can tolerate it.
However, do not try this unless you are sure you are able to tolerate butter.

Some brands of mixed (pie) spice contain gluten. If in doubt, make up your own jar with single, unadulterated spices, seal and store.

Index of Recipes

Index

cumin seed and rye bread 244
custard, ginger 133

dark ginger cake 220
date:
    and pecan muffins 252
    and walnut muffins 255
double chocolate chip:
    ice-cream 176
    muffins 254
double sticky gingerbread 209
duck with thyme and bacon 86
dumplings 71

Earl Grey tea loaf 223
Easter Simnel cake 231
elderflower and gooseberry cream 172
English scones 257
Eve's pudding, pear and blackberry 117
exotic pea purée 29

festive apple and mincemeat meringue 131
figs, baked 154
flapjacks:
    coconut and cinnamon 202
    low-fat ginger 204
    sesame 203
fondant Cape gooseberries 238
French apple tart 144
fruit cake 224

gingerbread 209
glazed apricot sausages 92
gnocchi with walnut and lemon sauce 41
greengage and almond tart 110
grilled salmon on puy lentils 59
grilled scallops with sage and capers 57
grilled sea bass with orange and vermouth sauce 50

haddock and mushroom roulade 62
halibut on beetroot and cumin purée 51

honey:
    glazed turnips 32
    and rosewater roll 222
hot pear brownie 115
hummus 12

ice-cream:
    banana and pecan with damson coulis 181
    Christmas pudding 183
    coconut 178
    double chocolate chip 176
    lemon curd 179
    Marsala 122
    praline 180
    sherry 102
    stem ginger 177

jelly:
    clementine and orange 164
    cranberry and wine with grapes 165
Johnny cakes and maple syrup 261

kiwi sauce 141

lamb:
    dauphinoise 72
    fillet with black bean salsa 74
    orange stuffed 73
lavender summer pudding 137
lemon curd:
    cake 217
    ice-cream 179
lemons:
    tart 149
    and walnut fettuccini 76
lime meringue pie 107
low-fat creamy pasta 45
low-fat oriental pork 75

macadamia nut pound cake 225
mackerel pâté 19